Decoding

The Secret Language of Your Body

The Many Ways
Our Bodies Send Us Messages

MARTIN RUSH, M.D.

A Fireside Book Published by Simon & Schuster
New York London Toronto Sydney Tokyo Singapore

FIRESIDE
Rockefeller Center
1230 Avenue of the Americas
New York, New York 10020

Copyright © 1994 by Martin Rush, M.D.

Designed by Crowded House Design
Manufactured in the United States of America

10   9   8   7   6   5   4   3   2

Library of Congress Cataloging-in-Publication Data
Rush, Martin.
    Decoding the secret language of your body: the many ways
our bodies send us messages/Martin Rush.
        p.   cm.
    "A Fireside book."
    Includes index.
    1. Medicine, Psychosomatic—Popular works. I. Title.
RC49.R87   1994   94-3518
616'.001'9—dc20   CIP

ISBN: 0-671-87238-9

To Walter Havighurst, beloved
professor and mentor, who taught
us to love our native language and
to appreciate its majesty and
beauty.

ACKNOWLEDGMENT

Dr. Milton Rosenbaum was formerly Chairman of the Department of the Albert Einstein College of Medicine, Yeshiva University in New York City, and is currently visiting Professor of Psychiatry at the University of New Mexico in Albuquerque. His thoughtful observations and supportive comments about the manuscript are deeply appreciated. Some of his suggestions made me rethink parts of the chapters, and his rich teaching experience helped to inject a note of confidence into what might have been for me doubtful ideation in several places.

Dr. Henry Lederer was Dean of Students and Professor of Psychiatry at Georgetown University School of Medicine in Washington, D.C. He had formerly been a Professor of Psychiatry at the College of Medicine of the University of Cincinnati. His encyclopedic knowledge of the literature of psychiatry rendered his comments and suggestions extremely helpful to me in preparing this manuscript. His death on January 4, 1994, was a great personal loss to me and his many other friends and colleagues.

Beginning in 1990, my fellow members of the medical staff at Middletown Regional Hospital have displayed a uniformly helpful and interested attitude about this project. At times they have buoyed my spirits and helped maintain my enthusiasm when it flagged. Many of them responded generously when I called them at odd times about fine points of their specialties, and so their influence upon the writing of this book has been profound. I thank all of you for your help—occasionally, the process felt as though it were a group effort, and I was enriched thereby. Despite your helpful input, the opinions expressed here are in no way your responsibility and are not meant as a reflection of the views of any of you as individuals or as a group.

C O N T E N T S

Part One
WHISPERS FROM THE BODY

Part Two
LOUDER CRIES FROM THE BODY

Part Three
WOMEN'S BODIES SPEAK THEIR MINDS

Part Four
SCREAMS FROM THE BODY

INTRODUCTION

I live and work in a high hazard area—for psychiatrists, that is. In my small midwestern town, the survival rate for psychiatrists is very low. Perhaps it is because there is a high level of good mental health in our town. In any case, a lot of people who live here seem to get along fine without ever seeing a psychiatrist.

When I came to town, I was the first and only psychiatrist. Over the last thirty-one years, I have seen fifteen psychiatrists come, open offices, finally close them, and depart. The fact that I am still here is probably not due to any particular merit on my part, but simply that this is my town and being very busy is not my highest priority.

I don't describe myself as a very successful physician volumewise, because I have never had a waiting list of longer than a week or so. My patients have learned that if they need to talk to me right away, I can usually work them into the schedule the next day or soon thereafter. I encourage people to avoid high-pressure situations, and that seems more comfortable for me as well. Perhaps in that way I am successful, because my life is comfortable, and it works for me.

As of this writing, my office out on the farm is the only full-time psychiatrist's office that has been here in our small midwestern town for more than a year. As it is, I'm never quite sure whether my patients come to see me or to enjoy the peaceful atmosphere of our little woodsy farm here on the edge of town, presumably, both. It is very pleasant to sit here in my office in the barnyard and look out at the woods and the seedling spruce tree I planted a hundred yards away, which is now about thirty feet tall.

One of the advantages of not being too busy is that it has given me the opportunity to approach my practice with more leisure and with time to think about the relationship between physical illness and emotional stress.

As a former family practice physician, part of my attention is always tuned to mention of my patients' physical illnesses as well as their emotional problems. Although I uniformly refer them for treatment of their physical illnesses to my former colleagues, a part of my thought processes is always trying to find a connection between their emotional state and their physical symptoms.

I left my family practice after five years, turning it over to my two partners with whom I had been working, to go back to school to study psychiatry. I remember that one of my colleagues bespoke the sentiment of many of my fellow physicians, "My gosh, Martin, why are you giving up the practice of medicine to go back and study witchcraft?" This may sound like an old-fashioned feeling to people in New York and Los Angeles, but here in Middletown, Ohio, even the medical community still has a few physicians who approach psychiatry with some suspicion, even in the nineties.

For the first years that I was back at the university, I sometimes wondered why I had given up the fulfilling role of the family doctor who delivered the babies, took care of the children and adults, and tried to ease the passing of the elderly. It was a wonderfully satisfying existence. I was proud of being their doctor, and my patients seemed to like me.

But I had to go back to the university to study psychiatry and to try to figure out why they got sick when their mothers-in-law moved in, their unmarried daughters got pregnant, or other stressful things happened to them. My obsessive puzzle-solving curiosity wanted answers.

After finishing my residence, I returned to my hometown to resume practice but now as a psychiatrist. Frequently, in the course of their therapy, my patients would mention a concomitant physical illness.

Formerly, in my role as family physician, I would have

simply asked them, "When did your (physical) illness begin?" In my role as psychiatrist, I began to ask them, "What was going on at the time you began to notice you felt bad?"

At first, most of them would say, "Nothing." However, as I learned with them how to carefully go back over their tapes of the events leading up to the illness, together we discovered an interesting fact. If they became ill, almost invariably we would find that the illness was preceded by some troubling event. Something had happened to disappoint them, or someone had bawled them out or hurt their feelings. Most often, they had blocked it out almost as soon as it happened because it was unpleasant. But their bodies, not being able to block things out, responded with illness.

Most of the time, there seemed to be an event associated with every illness, from headache to cancer, although many times, I wasn't clever enough to discover the precipitant.

As my patients had more therapy and became increasingly aware of how they were feeling, they learned to talk about their emotions before they built up steam. They didn't get ill so often. Patients who stayed in therapy for a year or more would wonderingly report that this was the the first year they could remember when they hadn't taken any antibiotics for frequent colds or had gotten through their allergy season without taking any shots.

This scenario is, of course, well known to most psychotherapists. They know that as people get "healthier" emotionally, they don't get physically ill as often. The more we notice the emotional messages, the less the backlog of feelings builds up, and the less we get ill.

As my patients and I together explored the relationship between emotional events and physical symptoms, we also began to realize that very often physical symptoms could lead us to unnoticed emotions we were having but to which we weren't paying any attention.

Human beings, it seems, don't notice a lot of feelings because we don't like to admit that we are unhappy. If something happens that makes us sad, we tend to block the sad feeling out as if it hadn't happened. This is why so many of our feelings occur without our "noticing."

On the other hand, if we get a pain in the neck or a cramp in the stomach, we don't ignore it. We can't. Like E. F. Hutton, when the body speaks, everybody listens.

Gradually, my patients and I began to realize that many of the physical symptoms we experienced were trying to draw our attention to emotional messages that we hadn't acknowledged. We began to look at symptom-means-emotion and found that by paying attention to small, hitherto unnoticed physical signs, we became aware of a host of small straws in the emotional wind that had passed over us without our being aware of the feeling. If we could recognize a delicate, faint emotion as soon as it cast its dim shadow over us, we could head for shelter before the cloud became a cloudburst.

Certain personality patterns seemed to be consistently connected with certain illnesses, some of them serious, even fatal. And that is how I came to write this book—because it seemed important to share what my patients and I had discovered together.

Most of the mind–body concepts mentioned here are simply restatements of generally accepted psychoanalytic theory. Some are not. As you read them, you can weigh them in your mind and feelings to see if they feel right for you. This is their ultimate validation.

For every illness, there seems to be an unhappy event of such a magnitude that it exceeds the "credit limit" of the body, and it goes into illness, which is a sort of bankruptcy or inability to function.

The person who is ill is unable to force himself to get up and go to work. His business suffers. If he recovers, business is resumed, cautiously at first, and with increasing vigor if the recovery is complete. If he cannot marshal enough good feelings so that his body (and his mind!) can get back into the profit side of the ledger, he slides inexorably into a decline and dies. He must have joy and satisfaction, or he perishes.

Each time we become ill, it is likely that it was "caused" by some unhappiness or stress in our life. Perhaps it was a discouraging word from someone, either close to us like a friend or a relative or, if we are the sensitive type, even from a perfect stranger. It may have been one more disappointment in a series of disappointments. In any case, it made us feel bad, we couldn't handle it, and our body expressed this through discomfort, pain, or illness—in short, dis-ease.

In other words, for every illness there may be an unhappy event that precedes and precipitates it. Consciously, we may not be aware of just what the last straw is, but it can make us sick. How could it be? Why don't we notice when something unpleasant happens to us? Furthermore, how do our bodies get involved just because our feelings are hurt?

That's what this book is about. Together, we can explore what happens to the body when we don't pay any attention to negative things that happen to us. Also, we will discover how our bodies are involved in every feeling, so much so that it can make us physically ill or even cause us to die prematurely.

The more attention we pay to our feelings, the more likely we are to notice when we feel bad and "let the feelings out" so that we don't get sick. The body will give us hints, and if we examine them, we will know what to look for, learn to recognize our feelings, and let them out, thereby avoiding pain and illness. Though we may not consciously notice a feeling, the body always notices and keeps score. We may lie to ourselves, but our bodies will always tell us the truth if we learn how to read and decode its signals.

But what about germs? Where do viruses fit in? What about constitutional predisposition? What about hereditary forces? Of course these all play their part in the great drama of health and illness. Nonetheless, researchers are methodically tabulating evidence that unpleasant life experiences lower our resistance to the microorganisms that cause disease and even cancer. Unfortunately, we have difficulty believing that unhappiness, which cannot be exactly measured, photographed, or weighed, has this fundamental impact on the health of the human animal. But the evidence is accumulating as recorded in the annals of psychoneuroimmunology.

Let us consider the possibility that each disease has its own distinct cry or complaint that its owner cannot recognize by virtue of her life training, nor is she permitted by that same training to complain aloud. Therefore, her body, that faithful workhorse with no speech to let out its melancholy lament, expresses itself in the only avenue left to it. It hurts, it quits its usual job, and the person becomes ill.

Perhaps if the patient could acknowledge her hurt and recognize the source of the hurt, she could cry out, so that her body would not need to make the powerful statement of discontent and unhappiness and throw in the towel.

Here we will try to chronicle the shared attitudinal patterns of people who have certain illnesses or symptoms in common. Those of us who are subject to similar stresses may be able to avoid the minefield ahead that has destroyed our unhappy fellows if we can remember in which direction they were marching.

Unfortunately, some of these illnesses we suffer are irreversible and will proceed to their unhappy end no matter what we do or think. However, other illnesses are reversible, and if we are correct in our hypothesis that certain combinations of attitudes and stresses lead to a worsening of certain disease conditions, we can perhaps save ourselves from unnecessary grief and pain.

A word about the case histories. All of them are based on actual cases, usually melded together from several of them but altered to protect the identity of my clients.

In addition, I have included some of my own experiences that I have been able to handle, after a fashion, as a result of my own therapy. Thus perhaps, I can urge my clients to do as I do as well as do as I say.

DISCLAIMER

This is not, strictly speaking, a scientific book. Traditionally, scientific findings are statistically measured, reproducible, and verifiable by independent observers. Thus, the scientific community is understandably cautious about accepting the kind of anecdotal data readers will find here, because personal data tend to be biased by personal points of view. Having arrived at an opinion about a particular subject—in this instance, the mind–body connection—people, even professionals like myself, will tend to use or present data that support that opinion.

Still, it cannot be denied that experience counts for something, and the observations contained in this book are based on more than nine thousand group meetings and over forty thousand individual psychotherapy sessions. Obviously, it is quite possible to repeat an error of observation an infinite number of times, but allowing for that, it is also quite possible to perceive the truth the first time it is observed. Having openly acknowledged that much, I share the conclusions here, knowing that they remain to be substantiated or disproved by scientific methods. I share them because my own observations of the connection between the mind, the emotions, and the body are based on solid experience. I share them because they may be of use and help to the reader.

Some of the concepts here may be new to you, and I urge you to withhold your acceptance or rejection of these ideas at least initially. As I caution my own clients, there is no point in trying to accept or believe an idea unless it makes good sense to you.

I ask only that you consider this material with an open mind. After reading about the experiences of others, you may want to apply these theories to yourself. You may be able to verify the mind–body connections explored in these pages, and then again, you may not. Should these ideas seem illogical, inappropriate, or unlikely to you, then obviously they are not going to work for you, and as every scientist knows, even the best ideas are useless if they don't work.

If you do find a connection or response to the ideas presented here, so much the better. My patients and I have found the ideas in this book to work over the years. Only you will know if they work for you.

Keep in mind also that scientific research must have new ideas to research and validate. Even the most dedicated researchers need some direction in which to proceed. And if enough observers like you and me and my patients agree that a premise makes sense, careful research can then subject that premise to thorough scientific analysis.

Some of the observations here are already part of accepted theory in psychosomatic medicine. Other messages from the body have long been accepted as part of the folklore that has come down to us through history, the kind of popular wisdom that stands the tests of time. The original observers of certain human behaviors certainly knew what they were doing. But the professional literature, including the burgeoning field of psychoneuroimmunology, have not, as far as I know, addressed many of the concepts described in this book.

A word about so-called psychosomatic illness: Many people, even some physicians, use the word interchangeably with *imaginary* illness. That is an error. Psyche + soma = mind + body. Hence, we have the word *psychosomatic*. Although folklore tells us that the notion of a mind–body connection is not entirely new, it is an idea that is slowly gaining increasing support both in the scientific and therapeutic communities. Many believe that the vast majority of illnesses occur because the mind (or emotions) adversely affect the functioning of the body, resulting in both minor disorders and major ones, such as infections, inflammation, neoplasm (cancer), and calculi formation (kidney stones, gallstones, and the like). Some of the processes by which these disorders can occur and their connection to the workings of the mind and emotions are discussed in this book.

The emotions felt in the body and transmitted to the consciousness in the form of physical symptoms are often so vague and ephemeral that we are not even aware of experiencing emotion at all. Whereas some people seem almost genetically preprogrammed to recognize most of their emotions, even the most transient, others are not. Still, most of us get better at it as we increase our awareness and think about our emotions, as often happens in therapy. Much of the material contained in these pages consists of observations made by myself and my clients in the course of therapy. I have protected their confidentiality here by altering the signature aspects of their stories. What has not been altered is the recurrence of the various phenomena of these connections seen so often by myself and my patients that we have mutually accepted the truth of the relation of certain emotions with certain physical symptoms as self-evident.

Though these observations have not been scientifically tested in the traditional sense, they have been proven to be valid by the grateful individuals who have lost their troublesome physical symptoms when they find the ability to express with words and voice an emotion previously expressed in an uncomfortable body. I would hope then that each reader will examine his or her own feelings when these whispered messages come to consciousness in the form of physical symptoms. Thus, we may all participate in a traditional function of scientific research: observation and documentation, acting as widely scattered independent observers.

But it should be remembered that body messages, like dreams, are unique to each individual. Just as dream analysis books have a limited usefulness because of each person's ability to conceptualize events and emotions in a supremely idiosyncratic fashion, so does each person have the ability to do the same in physical manifestations of their emotions. One person responds to an emotion with a pain in the neck, whereas another experiences the urge to pass gas.

CAUTION: On no account use anything written here as a reason for not seeking prompt medical help for any symptom you may experience. Many of the symptom messages described here are part of serious and life-threatening illnesses and should not be ignored or neglected.

You may very well experience some kind of stomach discomfort because you want a particular kind of love and attention, but stomach discomfort can progress to a bleeding ulcer, hemorrhaging, and death if not promptly treated. If you are experiencing any symptom that bothers you, see your doctor and obtain proper treatment.

Alexander Lowen, in his description of bioenergetic principles, has written extensively on the cold extremities and their relationship to fear. I am pleased to gratefully acknowledge his help to me as one of his many students in raising my consciousness of my own and others' body messages.

I would ask readers also to note that throughout these pages I have used words such as *perhaps*, *maybe*, and *sometimes* in describing situations and observations. I have expressed myself in a conditional fashion simply to avoid being dogmatic. Like the blind men describing an elephant, I am well aware that my version of the truth is not the only one available. Physical illness is easy to observe, to calibrate, and to prove. When discussing emotion, on the other hand, it is far more difficult to quantify. Ask three individuals what jealousy, sadness, or fear is and you are likely to get three quite different, yet equally valid descriptions of that emotion.

Careful attention to your feelings will either support or disprove the ideas here and determine their usefulness to you. Time will either substantiate or negate these concepts. Yet despite the difficulties inherent in trying to identify and understand the emotions, we must continue to try, for they rule our lives.

As individuals learn to come to terms with and to more accurately read and understand their feelings, they can be free of symptoms and experience more joy in just being alive. Awareness of the mind and body connection will, I hope, enable each reader to avoid unhappiness and illness, which, if the observations you find here are correct, may well be the same thing.

QUIBBLE

Why Should I Bother to Listen to My Body?

Your body is constantly whispering, giving off signals that are not just about what goes on in the body, but what goes on in the mind. Aches and pains, twitches and twinges, burps and coughs—we all experience these things, but we are not all aware that these body signals can have meaning beyond the physiological process involved.

But no matter how you might quibble, protest, or argue, the fact of the matter is, your body never lies. It always tells the truth; it cannot help but do so. You may smile at your hostess when she asks if she should switch on the air-conditioning, you can assure her that the room is quite comfortable, but all the time your body will make you out to be a liar. The perspiration will continue to flow, the flush in your cheeks will redden, you'll get increasingly thirsty.

Social niceties aside, though, the problem of physical manifestations of discomfort can sometimes go deeper than pretended politeness. For some, unrecognized or suppressed emotions can manifest themselves in the body through chronic pain, annoying twitches, and even some very embarrassing, socially incorrect problems like involuntary belching or flatus.

The greater the repression, the greater the emotional pain, the more serious and insistent become the signals from the body. Many illnesses, perhaps most illnesses, can be traced to an event or series of events in the emotional life of the individual. Physical discomfort is a tangible expression of those things that make us uncomfortable or unhappy in our hearts and minds.

But, just as the body expresses emotions through discomfort, just as misery can manifest itself in outright disease or even premature death, so other signals from the body can point the way to identifying those things that make us, quite literally, "feel good" the positive emotions and experiences that increase our immune systems, improve our attitudes, and help to ensure our all-around well-being.

What's So Good About Knowing How You Feel? Doesn't Everybody?

The fact is, most people can tell when they're wildly happy or just plain miserable. Extremes of emotion are relatively easy to recognize. But for the most part, we do not exist or experience life in an extreme emotional state. Most of us are taught early on that expressing excess emotion is socially inappropriate behavior. "Children should be seen and not heard." "Big boys don't cry." "Young ladies don't shout." The list goes on and on. Having learned or been conditioned not to express emotion, most of us learn to suppress our feelings to the point where sometimes even we are no longer aware of how and what we are really feeling.

Thus, the signals of the body can provide some interesting and valuable insight into our emotions. Try as we will, it seems, repressed emotion cannot be made to simply go away. Even when banished from our conscious thoughts, a feeling will find expression. Often that means of expression is through the ever-present, ever-truthful physical body.

Is It Really So Important to Know What I'm Feeling? Why Bother?

Being aware of the workings of the mind and emotions and their effect on the physical body is important because greater awareness leads to greater chances for happiness and appreciation of life. If, for example, Mr. X is used to stifling feelings of depression and dissatisfaction because he hates his job, he may, without being aware of it, be equally adept at stifling the feelings of contentment and joy he experiences in the time he spends with his family. In trying to keep his emotions on an even keel to collect a paycheck, he has painted himself a flat emotional landscape of dull grays. Yet the emotions that Mr. X is so good at repressing are not actually repressed at all. Mr. X has high blood pressure; he has painful indigestion. The quality of his work performance deteriorates due to debilitating headaches; his family life suffers because of chronic exhaustion. Taken to its worst extreme, the case of Mr. X could land him in a hospital or worse—a cemetery.

However, when you listen to your body and realize it may be telling you that you are unhappy with what's going on, the realization empowers you. You are free to walk away from the bore at a cocktail party, you can avoid the oppressor, or change your seat in the restaurant. Your blood pressure will return to normal, your heart rate will slow down, your guts will unclamp and return to their normal digestive processes.

Take our poor Mr. X. He may not be able to change his job, but knowing that he is prone to blinding headaches and troublesome acid indigestion when turning in last-minute monthly reports to Client Y, he may come to recognize that his dislike of the monthly reports is really a personal dislike of the client. By examining those feelings, he can then decide how to cope with them: by speaking directly to Client Y, by speaking with his boss or a colleague about switching clients, or even by taking some of the pressure off himself by recognizing that the agony of doing the reports is due at least partially to his own procrastination. By compiling the reports in small increments over the cycle, he is spared the double stress of time constraints and concern over his own performance and having to deal with that obnoxious Client Y. He is able to collect his paycheck, go home, and enjoy his family without obsessing over the reports.

What Happens to My Body When I'm Unhappy?

Let's change the above example somewhat. Mr. X and Client Y now work in the same office and carpool to the city every day. They have both changed jobs and are now colleagues. Mr. X doesn't like Mr. Y any better than he did before, but circumstances have thrown them together, so Mr. X goes back to his old ways.

When Mr. Y launches, as usual, into a recital of his gifted child's latest accomplishment, he forces Mr. X into admitting that his own child, at age ten, has never even heard of trigonometry. The car pool has five highway exits to go before they even reach the city, and needless to say, Mr. X is experiencing stress.

His body tenses as if for the kill. His intestines contract, stopping the digestion of his breakfast, and Mr. X can feel the acid beginning to churn. His fists clench; he is conscious of the beginnings of a blinding headache taking shape behind his eyes. He listens to Mr. Y with a fixed smile on his face. His mind drifts back to the story of Beowulf from his college days, the scene where the warriors around the campfire listened to the minstrel until "at length they wearied of him and slew him." Ahh, thinks Mr. X, shifting uncomfortably in his seat, no such luck.

But What Can I Do?

You and our Mr. X have a number of alternatives to cope with the annoying Mr. Y or any similar situation. Mr. X can

• Endure his stories in silence with a fixed smile on his face.
• Stop the car and ask him to either shut up or get out and walk.
• He can stop the car and get out and walk himself.
• He can try to change the subject.
• He can invite the man to find another ride.
• He can wait until he gets to the office and complain bitterly about the blowhard Mr. Y to sympathetic colleagues around the water cooler.
• He can work up a mean imitation of Mr. Y and perform it for his wife until she collapses in helpless gales of laughter when he gets home that night.

The only unhealthy response is the first one. Never endure in silence if you don't have to, and never endure for any longer than necessary. Mr. X's fellow carpoolers were suffering, too, and trashing him around the water cooler could very well prove an enormous relief for everyone. Making fun of the situation, tactfully changing the subject, all are fine alternatives. The point is, you cannot store up your anger in your body. Let it out! Deposit the toxic waste this man has dumped on your morning in a safe place and get on with your day.

What's So Good About Being Happy?

It is true that most people don't place being happy on their top ten list of priorities. It's almost as if they feel that happiness is some sort of accident. But the ability to be happy can be cultivated and developed, just like any other human potential. So, learn to work at it. First, because it feels good to be happy, much better than it feels to be unhappy, and second, happy people are infinitely healthier than unhappy people.

Emotions have an effect on the immune system.

When you're happy, it kicks into high gear and fights off things like infection and cancer. Your joints operate more smoothly, your digestion is better, you'll sleep more peacefully. The happy person who is in touch with and aware of his or her emotions has more energy and may even live longer. Best of all, cultivating an ability to be happy will enable you to truly enjoy life instead of merely enduring it.

So begin cultivating your own talent for being happy and healthy by learning to listen to your body's early warning signals, both your own unique signals and some others that you may discover in this book. Work to avoid or off-load negative feelings as you would the plague and hopefully you will also avoid disease, discomfort, and pain.

BIG BRAIN—ASSET
OR LIABILITY?

If you take a look at your dog or cat, you will notice that their skulls slope back rather sharply just above their eye sockets. The human skull, on the other hand, rises upward from the brow ridge to accommodate the twin bulges we call the cerebrum. Those two meatball-shaped structures, the lobes, are what we usually think of when we speak of the brain.

There's no doubt about it: If humans had brains like dogs and cats, they would probably not ever need to see psychiatrists, for it is the uniquely large human brain that not only makes them more intelligent than other species, but helps to set them up for neuroses.

The lower, more primitive part of the brain is also very important. In fact, lower animals have a brain very similar to our lower brain, part for part. Yet, with this simpler organ, they still seem to exhibit the emotions that we designate in an anthropomorphic fashion as love, hate, fear, jealousy, contentment, loyalty, excitement, and sadness.

Big Brain as an Asset

It is that bulging cerebrum that helps to make us the master species on this planet. The relatively massive cerebral cortex permits us to solve in an instant problems that would bewilder a lesser species. We can remember facts and manipulate concepts in a way that Rover could never comprehend.

The fact that we are gifted with a bigger and better brain is what makes a process like psychotherapy possible. We can get outside of ourselves; we can examine our patterns of behavior in at least a relatively objective fashion. With time, we can see and solve the neurotic patterns and problems that bedevil us all. Lesser creatures can be retrained, but it is doubtful that they would gain insight from the experience or benefit in the way a human being would from the change in his or her behavior.

Big Brain as a Liability

Even a small child is able to leave his pet dog behind in the learning race. Young as that child's brain is, it is soon shown to be far superior to that of even a mature and highly intelligent dog. The child can comprehend, for example that his mother loves him, but that sometimes she treats him with impatience when she is annoyed at his father.

With his superior intelligence, even an immature human is eminently trainable—capable of learning two or even more things at once. Unfortunately, those learning experiences sometimes connect in illogical ways that can develop into what we call neuroses.

Because that child has superior intelligence, he is able to make cause and effect connections. He becomes apprehensive when his father comes home, because he has learned that that is when his mother is more impatient with him. His reflexes conditioned, his muscles may tense when he hears Dad's car in the driveway. He may also begin to be petulant and demanding of his mother's attention at this time to get her reassurance that she really does love him despite her annoyance with dear old Dad. Should this situation happen consistently, the child's conclusions are reinforced and a neurosis is born. The child may be uncomfortable and uneasy around the father from childhood to adulthood for reasons that have nothing at all to do with the father's feelings toward the child.

Our complex intelligence allows each of us to be more aware of the many different aspects of the situations, events, and relationships around us. When wrong connections are made, it can set up conflicts that nag and worry us in many unpleasant ways for the rest of our lives.

There's no doubt about it. Lesser species are less neurotic. Your dog or cat seems unable to comprehend, much less feel conflicted about, many of the situations that give us humans so much trouble. Issues of morality, like incestuous attraction, polygamy versus monogamy, fair play, or human and property rights, seem to cause Rover or Fluffy no trouble at all. Your pet doesn't worry where the money's coming from or care about the mortgage payment. Part of that is due to a simpler, less intelligent brain. Part of it is due to the fact that pretense, which plays such a large part in the development of human neuroses, is almost entirely absent from the average dog's or cat's behavior.

The "what you see is what you get" modus of a dog or cat is, in some ways, far healthier than the games and conventions of manners, civility, power, politics, and expedition that we are all forced to play in the courses of our lives. We place such heavy burdens of pretense on our behavior that we can frequently collapse from the burden.

We scurry to tidy up and comb our hair when the doorbell rings to reveal a neighbor we don't want to see. Not so with a small child or a dog or a cat. If they don't want to answer the door or chat with so-and-so, they go hide under the bed.

Just as a small child surpasses the dog or cat in intelligence, she also learns that it is necessary to pretend in order to function in human society. She learns that it isn't nice to go hide under the bed and weep whenever so-and-so drops by. Mom and Dad may very well admit straight out that they think the child has the right idea, but even though everyone feels the same way, the child is taught the workings of pretense when she sees that not only are Mom and Dad not acting upon their feelings, but they are insisting that she not act upon her feelings as well. Thus, as the child learns to pretend, she picks up a burden of pretense that can be the very bane of a human being's life on earth. The more we learn to pretend, the more neurotic we become.

Seen from another angle, lesser species lack the ability to do the kind of long-term planning that highly intelligent humans do. We lie awake at night worrying about money, the mortgage, the state of our bank accounts and stock portfolios. If Rover manifests a tendency to long-term planning, it is usually quite decerebrate, the result of instinctual built-in patterns. Rover may bury a soup bone for tomorrow, but he could very easily forget where or even that he has done so. He may be hungry, but he is less worried.

No human being can successfully rid herself of her higher intelligence and hope to live the neurosis-free, happy-go-lucky life of one of the lower animals. Once you've had the big-brain experience, you never go back. Still, it is important to recognize that this bigger brain, with all of its assets, has a double-edged potential. It gives us an almost unlimited ability to learn, while at the same time, what we learn can be mistaken, resulting in neurotic and even destructive behavior. Yet, if we have learned wrong, if this grand brain of ours has created neuroses, it is equally capable of being used to unlearn those mistakes, as in psychotherapy, and rid us of our more troublesome conflicts.

THE DUALITY OF EMOTION

Emotions are apparently not spontaneous or mysteriously caused actions. They are reactions—to events, thoughts, experiences, or other stimuli. When we have an emotional reaction, the connection between the body and the mind becomes more obvious when we notice that two things happen at once:

1. There is a conscious awareness of the emotion, that is, I feel angry.
2. Physical and chemical changes take place in the body itself.

When something makes you angry or feel threatened, a series of physical changes begins with the hypothalamus, a butterfly-shaped area near the middle of the underside of the cerebrum. It sits just above and on each side of the small grape-shaped pituitary gland, which dangles down below the lobes of the cerebrum. The pituitary is sometimes called the *master gland* of the body and has direct connections with the hypothalamus above it. The hypothalamus is thought to be one of the more prominent areas in the brain where we feel our emotions.

When the hypothalamus sends impulses to the pituitary, as in the case of a threat, the pituitary, in turn, sends impulses to the adrenal glands just above the kidneys. The adrenals, in their turn, produce chemicals called *catecholamines*, including adrenaline, which produce physical changes in the entire body. The blood pressure rises, the heart beats faster, hairs all over the body stand up, the guts go into spasm. The blood supply surges and increases to the large muscles that we use to either flee the situation or attack.

This mass response to perceived threat was first described by the American physiologist Walter Cannon, who referred to this type of response as the *fight or flight response*. This type of body reaction is mediated by a complex system of nerves generally referred to as the *sympathetic nervous system*.

On the other hand, when the body is feeling safe and nonthreatened, able to enjoy activities like sex, digestion, or peaceful contemplation, that group of reactions is mediated by a network called the *parasympathetic nervous system*, sometimes called the "housekeeping" system.

So as you can see, the body has basically just two modes of response: one for war and one for peace.

With every emotion, there is both a mental response and a physical response, but sometimes our feelings are so well disguised or obscured that we are simply unaware of them and fail to notice either the mental or the physical changes produced by the emotion itself. Even more often we become adept at blocking the mental or conscious awareness of our emotions, yet continue to experience a sometimes bewildering set of physical responses or problems without knowing why. That is why I focus on these physical signs—so that you may notice emotions that might otherwise escape your attention.

Why Don't We Notice Our Feelings?

Most of us fail to notice or adequately respond to our own emotions simply because we are taught not to. When babies are hungry, they cry. When toddlers feel neglected or afraid, they holler until someone takes notice. When children are happy, they laugh and jump up and down. Small children do not pretend; what they feel is what they show the world.

As we grow older, however, we gradually become conditioned to hide our emotions in order to function in society. We learn that temper tantrums don't get you that new toy, that we will be punished for kicking Granny in the shins when she made us eat our spinach. We learn that displays of emotion, however justified they may be, do not make the world turn in our particular direction. Although the lessons we learn may indeed be valid, such as not expressing anger in destructive ways, in fact they are lessons we often learn too well, thanks again to the workings of our complex intelligence.

How to Grow a Neurosis

These oft-repeated, constantly reinforced messages are then built into us: "Emotions are a character flaw, a weakness. Stifle your feelings, keep them under control. Better yet, ignore them. Never show unhappiness; don't complain. Don't be jealous; don't feel sorry for yourself. And don't be too happy either or pleased with yourself. Everyone will think you're showing off."

Because we are gifted with the big brain, we are clever enough to incorporate all those thou-shalt-nots into our patterns of thinking and behaving. With all that superior intelligence equipment, we are eminently trainable and by the time we reach early adolescence, most of us have lost much of that early emotional awareness that made us so spontaneous and healthy.

However, just because we lose our awareness of emotions does not mean we cease to respond emotionally. What can and does happen instead is that we respond to a wide variety of emotional stimuli in totally inappropriate ways. This is known as *neurotic behavior.*

Civilization Versus Mother Nature

In our natural, uncivilized state, we roar with rage when we're angry. Sadness makes us weep; jealousy makes us want what we do not have and dream up all sorts of ways to get it. As part of the human species, we are aggressive, violent, and unpredictable. There is a part in each of us, the emotional, uncivilized part, that demands release and expression. Clearly, Mother Nature, in giving us our passionate emotional capacity, did not mean for those things to be stored up in the body or the mind. Aggression, tears, and laughter are our natural means of release.

Still, noble as a savage might be, civilization comes in pretty handy. Most of us wouldn't be without it. Civil laws prevent us from getting overly aggressive with each other, whereas common law, like traditional concepts of right and wrong, have gone quite a long way in enabling all these savage, passionate natures to get along with each other and share a planet.

No matter how high our degree of civilization, however, we humans respond to emotional stimuli in physiological, even primitive ways. We simply do not express emotion in the same ways our primitive ancestors did. Civilization has imposed such restrictions on the expression of our emotions, and our awareness of them has become dulled and obstructed. Nonetheless, powerful, even primitive physical and emotional responses remain. If we don't fully understand the nature of those responses, as humans we sometimes cope by engaging in behavior that doesn't make sense or is simply inappropriate. This is called *neurotic behavior.*

If we desire to rid ourselves of these neuroses, we must find ways to get in touch with our forgotten or repressed feelings. On the other hand, if our emotions go unrecognized, the physical responses evoked by those emotions can go equally haywire, resulting in pain, disease, and even death.

This does not mean that we have to be uncivilized in order to be healthy. Knowing that you would like to haul off and slug an obnoxious person does not mean that you have to act it out to be emotionally and physically healthy. But recognizing the feeling, admitting it, and avoiding that person in the future can help you to avoid the physical discomfort that goes with repressed emotion—a pain in the neck, a sudden headache, or stomach discomfort.

Recognizing our feelings enables us to express them and expressing the feeling enables us to release that feeling from the body.

How We Emote with Our Bodies

Physiologists have known for years that we think and feel with our bodies. The mind and emotions are not separate from the body itself. Try this experiment: If you close your eyes and think about writing your signature, as you think of writing each character in your name, the muscles in your arm will be activated in the same order as if you were actually signing your name. They may even twitch so that you can feel it. Even if they do not twitch, a series of electromyograph tracings will show that your brain is sending faint commands to your hand and arm, just as if you were actually signing your name.

In the same way, if you feel a certain fear as you make your way to a business meeting, your body seems to experience the trip to the meeting in fantasy. As you imagine going through the door of the office building, your body will handle the anticipated unpleasantness by expressing it physiologically as a potential danger. Usually, this physical manifestation of fear or the feeling of potential danger will happen in the part of the body that encounters the danger first, namely, the feet that are taking you to this place you are afraid to go. To keep you from losing blood, the blood vessels in the skin of your feet will contract, leaving the skin cold. This physical manifestation of a feeling of dread is so common, the expression "cold feet" has become interchangeable with the idea of being afraid or apprehensive.

The body can also conceptualize current or anticipated events in the same way it might have in an earlier stage of development, like infancy. We can anticipate a new car with the same enthusiasm that an infant would physically anticipate a warm bottle of milk. If we don't get that car, the stomach might contract painfully as if we were hungry. Likewise, if we experience something that is more than we ever hoped to have, that represents some kind of overgratification, we may feel the need to vomit, to rid ourselves of that which seems too much.

There's no getting around it; the body experiences emotion simultaneously with the conscious or even unconscious mind. To reduce our inappropriate, or neurotic, responses to those emotions, we must become more aware of how and what we are feeling, minute by minute.

Perhaps the way to that greater self-awareness is to pay closer attention to the body itself and the signals it constantly broadcasts. If the body says, "I feel bad," listen to it. Try to notice what is making you unhappy and remove yourself from that situation if you can. If you are unable to do so, complain—let out your unhappy or negative feelings. Whine, complain, yell, scream, gnash your teeth, or pound a pillow. Though it sounds a bit simplistic, the simple act of expression can prevent you from accumulating the toxins and developing the symptoms that left unattended can lead to disease.

Listening to your body and learning what it is trying to tell you will not only improve your health and the quality of your life but can also be a fascinating and intriguing adventure. As you become more adept at identifying your own feelings and expressing them, you will also find yourself more sensitive to others, more easily able to relate and encourage them to express themselves. It is an unwritten law of the universe that like attracts like. Unhappiness and other negative emotions attract the same from people around you and provoke negative and unhappy physical manifestations of that state of being. By the same token, contentment and happiness brings out like responses in not just your own body, but in the people around you. If you are happy, others will feel good in your presence. The better you feel physically, the easier it is to be happy. The happier you are, the easier it is to make that happy condition a way of life and health.

Whispers

from the Body

INTRODUCTION

To be really alive it seems important to be alert to our feelings. To be really healthy, it is equally important to be aware of those signals from the body that can result from our failure to notice or acknowledge our feelings.

The following part contains signals from the body that might best be classified as "whispers" that are designed to bring your attention to emotions you might otherwise miss. These might seem at first glance somewhat inconsequential, but as discussed later on in the book, it can be a mistake to ignore even moments of feeling as they have a way of adding up in the body's computer. The impact of even little feelings has a way of accumulating when ignored or repressed and may even be the reason you get ill when you do.

These whispers are all fairly benign, at least at the outset. But to notice them is the first step on your way to a greater awareness of your feelings and the body's signaling system as a whole. Think of the whispers as an introduction to the body–mind connection. Listen to their secrets, and see if the descriptions here feel accurate to you. Greater awareness of your body and emotions can lead to an improvement in the quality of your life as a whole, and that's what we're hoping to achieve.

THE BLUSH

The blush is one of the best known and most widely recognized signals from the body. Generally speaking, when a person blushes, it is a clear indication that they are embarrassed in some way. But a blush can mean other things, too, as we shall see later on.

The physiology of the blush involves the network of tiny blood vessels that lie just under the surface of the skin. These tiny veins, or capillaries, act in response to both external and internal stimuli. They act almost like radiators, expanding and contracting to heat and cool the body as required. When the capillaries contract strongly, they seem to burrow deeper into the skin. Body heat is held in, the blood goes to the muscles and other organs, and the skin has a blanched appearance.

When these little blood vessels expand, they seem to bring blood closer to the surface of the skin, cooling the body down. In this case, the skin turns red or fiery pink, and we feel warm as the body works to let off excess heat.

Most of the time, the capillaries lie just far enough below the surface to give the skin its normal color. When physiology joins with psychology, the process of blushing goes like this:

1. The mind or emotions decide we want something. In turn, this sends a message to the body to get ready to go after it—to get ready to fight, if necessary. The blood vessels in the skin contract slightly, sending the blood to muscles; perhaps there is muscle tension or adrenaline rush, as we discussed in the fight or flight response.

2. For whatever reason, we then become aware of the possibility that other people (real or fantasized) would not approve of our desires.

3. Feeling trapped between what we desire and the opin-

ions and approval of others, the mind sends the body into a "cool it" mode. Having encountered obstruction to our desire, we feel trapped. The body, unable to pursue its inherent desire to fight or flee, then "surrenders." The muscles relax; the capillaries expand, bringing blood to the surface, coloring the skin, and we blush. The person who is blushing feels an accompanying warmth, beginning at about the level of the heart. The flush climbs upward at varying rates to the neck the face and even the scalp area.

Naturally in therapy, both client and therapist encounter many occasions for blushing. However, my favorite story about this phenomenon involves a trip I took to Japan several years ago.

In Kyoto, the lovely old former capital city, my wife and I were busily exploring some back streets away from the glitzier tourist shopping areas. We were feeling self-consciously superior, assuring ourselves that we were getting to know the "real" Japan.

We were intrigued by the dark inconspicuous little shops that lined the streets and fancied they were patronized by the local citizens. When my wife went into a used clothing store to look at some faded but elegant old kimonos, I wandered down the street and paused at the window of a small, drab shop that seemed to specialize in carved bamboo objects, whistles, tea stirrers, tubular boxes, and the like. My attention was drawn to a small tubular box containing two delicate little carved spoons, about the size of matchsticks, one natural in color, the other burned or stained black.

Inside the store, the proprietor and another man were having tea together across the counter. They rose politely when I entered and I indicated in my inadequate Japanese that I would like to examine the box and its contents. The owner removed it from the window and placed it on the counter with a slight bow. When I asked the purpose of the little spoons, the owner indicated somewhat uncomfortably that they were for the removal of earwax. When I asked why they were of different colors, he explained in English that was only slightly better than my Japanese that one was for the woman, the other, for the man.

I couldn't help but notice his discomfort, and my curiosity was piqued. I asked for more specific information about these curious gender-linked grooming aids. The merchant glanced to his friend for help, but his friend only shrugged and remained silent. Finally he explained in halting English, "She do to him. He do to her."

At this revelation, both he and his friend blushed beet red and avoided my eyes. Sharing their discomfiture because I wanted the little box with the spoons, I blushed myself but wasn't quite sure just what the implications of my purchase of it might be. I paid for the box and left the store.

I've never been able to find out the rest of the story of the little earwax spoons or why those men blushed at my questions, so clearly uncomfortable. Were they part of some exotic aphrodisiac ceremony? Were they considered some sort of marital or sexual aid? Were the men embarrassed by my ignorance? I'll never know.

If you blush a lot, you may wish to consider that perhaps you want something (maybe quite often) that you're not sure you should want or that others think you should have. Caught in the act of wanting, you may be feeling guilt or embarrassment. You can't fight and you can't flee, thus your body goes into a back-pedaling mode. Your capillaries expand, your tense muscles weaken; in effect, you surrender, through your embarrassment, to other's opinions.

One correspondent has told me she invariably blushes when she gets up before a group to make a presentation. Presumably this means she wants something from the group: their approval, their acceptance of her presentation, whatever. She fears rejection or embarrassment and begins to blush uncontrollably.

If this woman could learn to voice her misgivings, on the other hand, she could begin her speech by simply saying straight out that she is always nervous before a crowd. She can even mention her blushing if she wishes. Chances are, her audience will be disarmed by her candor and empathize with her situation. Having gotten that out of the way, she will no longer feel that she has anything to hide, and so her body will have lost the need to blush.

In a way, this is like throwing yourself on the mercy of an adversary. By voicing or admitting your misgivings—verbal surrender—you will free your body from its need to surrender physiologically.

THE COUGH

Have you ever been in the middle of a conversation only to find yourself possessed by an unexplained fit of coughing? You know you don't have a cold, postnasal drip, or an allergy, yet for some unexplained reason there you are, all but choking. Then, when the subject is changed or the conversation moves on, the cough abruptly subsides.

What were you thinking about before that cough began? Very often, when a thought rises to consciousness, when the words to convey that thought are formed and ready to be voiced, you change your mind and suppress those words at the last minute. Instead of letting the words out, you literally swallow them, and you begin to cough.

This seems to be the mind–body process connected with the cough:

1. You are about to say something, change your mind, and literally swallow your words instead of letting them out.
2. To get ready to swallow, your salivary glands secrete a small bolus of saliva to help lubricate the material to be swallowed. That lubrication helps whatever it is to go down the food pipe, or esophagus, more easily.
3. In the act of swallowing, the semirigid windpipe is lifted upward to let the swallow package pass over it into the esophagus and down into the stomach. This process is easily observed in the action of a man's Adam's apple as it moves up and down.
4. When you are about to speak and change your mind, however, the windpipe is open to let air in and words out, and the saliva you secrete to swallow goes into the open windpipe.
5. The reflexive protective mechanism kicks in as you feel saliva going into your windpipe and you begin to cough in order to blow it back out again.

6. You can't talk when you are coughing, so you very literally choke on your own words.

The body never lies. Chances are, when you choke up on something, it means you have mixed feelings about a subject, a conversation, or your own thoughts on a particular subject. The body signal is letting you know that you are undecided about bringing your thoughts and feelings up and out into the open in the form of words or swallowing them and keeping those thoughts and feelings to yourself.

Brad L., a forty-six-year-old economics professor who was planning a move to the country with his family, was relating in therapy an encounter he'd had with a real estate salesman who was showing him several small farms.

"We were riding down the road, and I mentioned that I had once heard that for about ten thousand dollars a person could bribe a dishonest state planning board employee and find out where they were going to run a new highway. I told the salesman I had heard the real estate people could then figure out where the cloverleafs would lie and buy up the land from farmers very cheaply. In a year or so, the land could be resold to developers to put in shopping centers, motels, and restaurants, making the real estate people a bundle in profit.

"Well, this fellow was just driving along, not saying anything, but he began to cough so hard he almost had to pull off the road. I was afraid he'd choke to death. His face was almost purple, he was coughing so much.

"I don't know if he knew somebody who was doing this, if he was doing it himself, or if he was simply mad because he hadn't thought of the scheme himself. He never said anything, just blew his nose and nodded. Maybe he thought it was a bad thing to make a profit that way but really wished he could do it—he never said a word.

"But I never bought any of the farms he showed me. His heart just didn't seem to be in it after that."

The Cough 49

Virginia T., a thirty-four-year-old industrial designer, another client, was relating a dream she'd had a few nights previous to our appointment.

"A strange man came jogging through my bedroom early in the morning. He came leaping through the open window, running with long strides right past my bed. I wasn't afraid, though, because my husband was out of town and I was alone."

She paused, and as she recognized what she'd just said, she colored and began to cough uncontrollably. After her fit of coughing had subsided, she managed a small laryngitic squeak: "Boy," she said. "Talk about choking on something. I didn't know what I was saying until I heard it come out."

Needless to say, Virginia's libidinal impulses had jumped to the forefront, and she had striven unsuccessfully to choke them back down. After she'd gotten her breath, she began to laugh ruefully.

"I guess I do have some impulses that get away from me. Well—almost!"

Again, the cough is a signal from the body that you have mixed feelings about something. In Virginia's case, her cough was telling her that she had impulses that she wasn't entirely comfortable admitting. She was simultaneously responding to and suppressing a libidinal impulse, resulting in that telltale cough.

So the next time you have an unexplained cough that is unrelated to a physical disorder, check it out. Examine and express, if you can, your mixed feelings—those words and thoughts you were trying so hard to swallow.

GOOSE BUMPS

When you experience goose bumps, you are experiencing a thrill. The thrill itself can be either pleasant or unpleasant in nature; the signals your body gives off are the same.

Physiologically, goose bumps are part of the fight or flight response, involuntary contractions of the small muscles in the skin around the hair follicles. The original purpose of the goose bump phenomenon is still seen in the animal kingdom. When an animal encounters a sudden threat, an unexpected noise, or is otherwise startled, the animal's body goes into the fight or flight mode that usually includes a sudden erection of the hairs on its body, fluffing out the fur, to make the animal look larger and more formidable to an approaching enemy. Fur can also fluff up in response to cold, providing insulation for the body against sudden drops in temperature, and certainly some goose bumps are simply a response to environmental conditions. But for a more domestic example of the fight or flight aspects of goose bumps, take an ordinary dog or house cat. When threatened, the hair rises on its body, particularly along the spine and around the ruff, or neck (in order to make it more difficult for a predator to go for the animal's throat).

People can experience goose bumps in any variety of circumstances. For example, if you come into a darkened house at night and move about without turning on the lights, a sudden noise may give you goose bumps. A creaking floorboard may make you catch your breath, make your heart seem to skip a beat, and cause goose bumps to break out along your arms and scalp.

On the other hand, you may experience goose bumps due to a thrill of pleasure. In this case, it is almost as if the body is saying, "This is too much! I can't believe I'm experiencing this. This is so wonderful someone is sure to try and take it away from me! I must be in danger."

Of course, when you get goose bumps, only you can tell if you're experiencing a threat or a thrill. Perhaps there is an element of danger in either case. Take the following example.

Kelley R., a thirty-seven-year-old receptionist who had come into therapy to increase her capacity for pleasure, described the first time she met her daughter's fiancé.

"Lonnie said to me, 'Mom, I want you to meet Bill.' Well, I want you to know, I turned around and was face-to-face with the handsomest man I've ever met! He made my head swim! Of course, I tried not to let it show, but if he marries Lonnie and is around all the time, I'm in trouble. I feel like a high school girl every time he's around.

"I really do have to keep reminding myself that I'm the mother of the bride, not the bride-to-be. Bernie, my husband, likes him, too, but not like I do, let me tell you. I hope he hasn't noticed the effect Bill has on me. Lord, I can't get over the way he makes me feel. I even dreamed about him last night. Will you look at these goose bumps on my arms?"

Clearly, Kelley was experiencing the kind of thrill that had an obvious element of danger attached. Her attraction to her future son-in-law was indeed a kind of pleasure, but its forbidden quality held obvious elements of danger as well.

In addition to the fact that the body never lies, it is curious to note that the body has a long memory as well. Sometimes an individual will get goose bumps simply by remembering an incident they found unusually thrilling or threatening.

Olga N., a fifty-one-year-old professor of music, recounted seeing the great Judy Garland just a few months before her death. As a young girl, Olga had been profoundly influenced by Judy's rendition of "Over the Rainbow" in the movie *The Wizard of Oz*.

"I'd been a fan of hers for most of my life, so you can

imagine how I felt when I finally got to see her in person on a magnificent big stage in Las Vegas.

"She'd been out of sight for many months, taking the cure for alcohol and drugs, or at least that was the rumor. But when she walked out on that stage, it was like a miracle.

"She kidded with the crowd, things like 'You didn't think I'd make it back, did you?' or 'You didn't think my legs would look this good, huh?' Everybody—all of us there—we loved it. She did a little soft-shoe, got a bit winded, and sat down on the edge of the stage to get her breath. She asked a man at one of the front tables to share his glass of water with her. I bet he's got that glass somewhere in a display case to this day!

"Finally she asked the crowd what song they'd like to hear. From every corner of the room, with one voice, the crowd roared 'Over the Rainbow'!

"The hall was hushed for a long moment. Judy Garland, who may have sensed by then that she didn't have too many months left, clasped her hands in front of her and stared down at the floor.

"There were tears in her eyes when she raised her face to the crowd and began to sing. There were tears in our eyes, too. Here was this incredibly gallant woman going on with the show no matter what. She had taken a beating, but she wasn't beaten. Not yet.

"By the time she finished that song, tears were rolling down my face. I was sobbing; goose bumps were all over my body. The whole crowd held its breath to hear that last note. We screamed and shouted, and everyone threw the flowers from the tables to the stage at her feet. She just stood there, loving her audience the way they loved her."

Olga looked down at her arms when she was done with the story. "Look," she told me. "I've got goose bumps all over again; just telling you about it. I'll never forget that night. Not as long as I live."

Hopefully, Olga's goose bumps won't forget either,

and the joy and excitement she experienced that night will never leave her.

Goose bumps are yet another piece of evidence of the body–mind connection and of how the emotions affect physiology. In fact, your body may notice how you feel even before you can put that feeling into conscious thought. Similarly, if a memory triggers goose bumps, it may be a signal that some event or occurrence had a bigger impact on you than you may have originally thought.

THE SNEEZE

The sneeze has been called an orgasm of the face. It is one of the body signals that merits great attention because an unexpected sneeze is often an indication of having encountered an unexpected pleasure. Once you experience and become aware of the sneeze–pleasure connection, it becomes a friend you're always ready to welcome back.

Tanya G., a thirty-four-year-old waitress, sat in my office, wringing her hands as she talked.

"So, he's been seeing her for the past six months and seeing Connie, too, who's been divorced for the past year. There he is, keeping both of them on the string and I never even suspected. I feel like a fool.

"I thought he really loved me. He tells me all the time he's glad he's married to me. I mean, I knew he liked women, and that they always flirted with him, but I never dreamed he was cheating on me!"

Tanya was quiet for a few moments, gazing out the window.

Finally, she spoke again. "I wonder how he'd like it if he came home and found me in bed with somebody else. Our friend Howard has been hitting on me the past few times I've seen him. I'd never give in of course, but—"

All at once, she sneezed. She reached for the box of tissues, which is a standard piece of equipment in a psychiatrist's office. Before she could get one, she sneezed again. Smiling, Tanya grinned at me roguishly. "I guess I like that idea."

"The sneeze says it all," I answered.

The ancients saw the sneeze as an evil omen. Thucydides said sneezing was a crisis symptom of the great Athenian plague. Saint Gregory has been credited with originating the custom of saying "God bless you" after someone sneezes, the story being that he began to do so during a pestilence in which sneezing was a mortal symptom. The Romans took up the practice with the usual exclamation of *Absit Omen*, whereas the German *Gesundheit* is a wish for the good health of the sneezer.

Physiologists have pointed out that at the moment of sneezing, the pressure inside the rib cage is suddenly increased to the point where the regular action of the heart is stopped for a moment. Perhaps the ancients sensed this phenomena and so regarded it as evil.

Of course, as time went on, people began to recognize the pleasurable sensation of sneezing and even to induce it. The widespread practice of taking snuff was hugely popular in the seventeenth, eighteenth, and well into the nineteenth centuries.

But the fact is, people sneeze very suddenly in response to their emotions as well as to physical causes like colds, allergies, pepper, or snuff. Physiologically, the sneeze is usually a response to noxious substances in the nasal passages. In the absence of such substances, the nasal passages sometimes seem to partake in a fantasied response to pleasure: the sweet smell of success or when a happy thing is either present or imagined. It is as though your nasal passages are thrilled. The hairs inside the passages stand on end, it tickles, and you sneeze.

Not only do humans sneeze to express pleasure, other animals do as well. Dogs and cats sneeze in expression of their pleasure at extra attention, and horses sneeze as well. The domestic animals' response of the sneeze as an expression of pleasure is well documented. It is possible the phenomenon also exists in the wild, but I am unaware of this.

When you sneeze, look for a good feeling first rather than assuming you're coming down with something. It is probably there somewhere. For example, people have reported regular postcoital sneezes or sneezing during the initial phases of sexual arousal. Others will walk out of a dark building into the brilliant sunshine and sneeze. This is sometimes referred to as a *sun allergy* but is more likely to be a response to the pleasure they experience from the warmth and light of the sun. The pleasurable effects of bright light have been recognized and documented, even resulting in the manufacture of mood-elevating lights, which provide a strong daylight intensity of light in stores and offices, replacing those endless rows of fluorescent tubes. They have been shown to improve both mood and productivity.

Pamela G., a forty-one-year-old bank teller, had worked with me for months to try and discover the reasons for her own self-defeating pattern of repeatedly taking up with punishing, deprecating men. "They're never like that in the beginning," she would complain. "It's just that once I get to know them and trust them, they start treating me like dirt. They call me bad names, say I'm stupid, and even slap me around."

She had come to the point where she was aware that each of these men was created in the image of her hostile and angry father, who had consistently abused her for the smallest of transgressions, calling her "another goddamn stupid bitch like your mother."

As doctor and patient, we had been over and over this material, and she claimed she understood her feelings but would then go right out and establish yet another relationship with yet another abusive man.

Then, one day in our session, she thoughtfully reported a long-forgotten incident from her childhood. Her father grabbed her, roared with rage, and pulled out his belt to beat her across the back.

"And do you know," she told me in a low voice, "I remember I felt a real surge of joy. There he was yelling at me and beating me, but it didn't hurt at all. All I could think about was that I had finally gotten his attention—all of his attention—and that he wasn't ignoring me like he did the rest of the time. It felt so good, just having the attention. Do you think that's the way I feel with men? That I don't care if they abuse me as long as I've got their attention?"

I regarded her soberly, trying to keep a lid on my own elation. All the months of work had finally paid off. She had made the connection. It might still be a long time before she could incorporate it into her behavior, but she'd made the connection at long last! I wanted to grab her and dance around the room, I wanted to send out for champagne. Instead, I nodded soberly. Suddenly, I sneezed.

She glanced at me. "You liked that, huh? Boy, I bet you thought I'd never get it."

Lorena T., another patient, took issue with me on the significance of the sneeze. "I've always heard that if you sneeze when you meet someone, it means you're allergic to them. Like this man I met at a party last week. I knew immediately I didn't like the guy. The moment we were introduced, he said, 'Charmed, I'm sure.' It was really affected, you know, pretentious. Then I sneezed, and he asked, 'Is your cold contagious?' Honestly, I felt like slugging the guy. I said I figured I must be allergic to something and looked him right in the eye. He didn't turn a hair, just stood there smirking."

"How did you feel about him?" I asked.

"I thought he was arrogant and insufferable. You could just tell he was the type who thought he was God's gift. And can you believe it? He got my phone number from the hostess and called me last night. Said he wanted to take me to dinner at a place he knows I'd like. See what I mean? I met the guy once and already he thinks he knows what I like."

"What did you tell him?"

"I finally decided to go just to get him off the phone. Besides, I want another chance to let him know what a jerk I think he is."

Needless to say, I did not comment any further on the subject of her sneeze.

• • •

Why is the sneeze so important? I believe that if we can identify those things that cause us to experience pleasure, then perhaps we can prolong the experience and learn to cultivate those good feelings. As the adage says, *Carpe diem*, "Seize the day."

The more often we experience pleasure, the more unwilling we are to remain in our more routine states of feeling dull, inadequate, or unhappy. As we become more experienced in the world of positive feelings, the more necessary they become to us. Physiologically, we can benefit from pleasure because the experience of pleasure releases endorphins and encephalins from the brain. The immune system benefits from good feelings, and even the phagocytes, those scavenger cells that float around in our body fluids, proceed with more vigor as they move around and gobble up viruses, germs, and stray cancer cells.

So, sneezes are worth noting. They mean that there's a good feeling nearby, waiting to be acknowledged and, if at all possible, prolonged.

COLD HANDS AND FEET

Under certain conditions, the autonomic nerves that control the diameter of the arteries, and hence the blood supply to the fingers and toes, will cause those arteries and their tiny branches to contract, all but completely cutting off the blood supply to the extremities. The fingers or toes will then become white, numb, and cold.

This phenomenon is generally referred to as *Raynaud's syndrome* or *Raynaud's disease*. In relatively rare instances, it can be a manifestation of underlying systemic disorders or serious disease, but most of the time, cold, weak, or numb fingers seem to be an intermittent condition related to emotional conflicts. Though attacks usually last only a few minutes, they have been known to last hours or even days, to the extent that such attacks can permanently damage the affected areas.

What is the nature of the conflict that causes this phenomenon? The causes are as individual as the individuals affected by this disorder, but generally speaking, cold, weak, or numb fingers seem to be the body's way of expressing conflict over wanting literally "to reach out and touch" something but suppressing that impulse to the point where touching or grabbing something becomes impossible, because the sense of touch itself is temporarily absent from the benumbed fingers. People who are afflicted with this disorder are frequently conditioned to "look and yearn, but don't touch." They are frequently more conscious of the rules and regulations than other people and more afraid to break those rules as well. They want the things we all want—the love, the promotion, the pleasure of recreation—just as much as anyone else but don't feel they deserve to get it.

Similarly, we all know the expression cold feet, which has become synonymous with fear, or, more specifically, the kind of fear that comes with wanting something and being afraid of it at the same time. Brides and grooms are famous for cold feet—they want to get married but are afraid to do so.

Another, more severe manifestation of the fear of reaching for what you want is known as *carpal tunnel syndrome*. With this disorder, the sufferer is literally and painfully prevented from getting her hands on what she wants, because pain in the wrists prevents the fingers from closing around anything at all.

In this instance, the effect is not due to the contraction of blood vessels in the hand. It is a progressive tightening of the ligaments in the wrist, like a too-tight watchband. In severe cases requiring surgery, some of the ligaments are severed in order to loosen the constriction in the wrist that causes the weakness in the hands and fingers. Such surgery may help, or it may not.

Traditionally, carpal tunnel syndrome is thought to be caused by certain systemic diseases or more frequently by occupations that require repetitive movements of the wrists, like those of typists or computer operators. Repetitive action is thought to cause a tightening of the ligaments, resulting in a progressive loss of function.

I have seen several cases of carpal tunnel syndrome in several of my patients, and always there is an underlying history of a "look but don't touch, much less take" conditioning. They seem literally unable to reach for those things they desperately want, such as a new house or a better job. Contrary to traditional thinking on the subject, the patients I have treated with carpal tunnel syndrome are not always in a job or a phase of their lives where the condition could be described as an occupational hazard. However, during the course of therapy, we have come to recognize the causes and nature of the fears that are holding them back, surgery has been avoided, and their grip, both their physical grip and their grip on themselves and their emotions, have improved dramatically.

If your hands or feet become numb, cold, or weak, consider your fears first. See if you can figure out what it is that you want but don't feel that you deserve. Think about it, talk about it, and the trouble in your fingers and toes will probably abate.

THE DRY MOUTH

In ancient China, there was a test for truth in the courtroom. The person testifying before the court was asked to hold a dry pebble in his mouth as he told his story. When he was finished, if the pebble was wet, he was presumed to be telling the truth. If it was dry, he was presumed to be lying.

The problem with the test, of course, is exactly the same problem as exists with today's polygraph tests. The stress of lying and the stress of simply being accused of lying can produce the same physiological responses.

Exactly how does the dry mouth fit into the body's master plan? As we have discussed, the body has two modes of operation: one for war—the fight or flight response—governed by the sympathetic nervous system, and one for peace, or housekeeping, governed by the parasympathetic nervous system. Depending on what's going on around you, the body can switch modes almost instantly.

Dry mouth is almost invariably an indication of nervousness or fear. When your mouth suddenly goes dry, your tongue sticks to the roof of your mouth, your breath quickens, and you may find it difficult to swallow. In short, your body has switched once more into a fight or flight mode of operation.

To win a fight or to escape with your life, your body is programmed to eliminate or put on hold all functions that are unnecessary for survival. Obviously, if you are fighting for your life, you are not eating, so who needs a moist mouth? The blood supply for the salivary glands is shut down, diverted to your muscles, and your mouth dries up.

Let's look at a couple of examples.

Milton T., a twenty-six-year-old securities salesman, frequently showed up for his sessions in tennis whites, lolling casually in a chair facing me as we talked.

"You know, Doc, I've noticed something interesting. Whenever I come to see you, as I pull into the parking lot, my mouth gets dry. No kidding, I could spit dust."

"How do you feel about coming here?" I asked him.

"Well, I really don't mind it. Most of the time, I sort of look forward to it, I guess. But at the same time, I am starting to think I dread it, too."

"Any idea why?"

"No. I mean, I'm not afraid of you. But I was thinking, it's the same kind of dry mouth I get when I have to hit Dad up for a loan. I just know how he's going to accuse me of being irresponsible—all the same old crap, even though he always gives it to me anyway. Come to think of it, maybe I am afraid of you! I used to get the same thing when I was a kid and they sent me to the principal's office!"

Margie L., a thirty-one-year-old married secretary, was an inveterate coquette and a compulsive adventuress with other women's husbands. She loved her own husband, Nathan, but as she roguishly complained, she was the kind of girl who just couldn't say no! She'd never been caught and had not told me about her hobby of bedding down with other women's husbands until I had been seeing her for well over a year.

"I'm sitting at a table eating lunch, and I look up and notice this guy is looking at me. I glance at him, glance down at my plate, and the next thing I know, he's standing at the table asking if he can join me. After that, it's all a kind of dance. I call Nate and tell him I'm working late and see the guy instead. I end up in a motel room with this guy I met at lunch.

"But when I pull into the parking lot at our apartment complex, my mouth goes completely dry. I swear, my tongue sticks to my teeth. Every time I go out with a new guy like this my mouth dries up like the Sahara Desert when I get home."

"What does Nate say when you come home late?"

"Nothing. He's usually watching the ball game. He waves, goes on watching. I go into the kitchen and get myself a glass of water."

"What are you feeling when you pull into the parking lot?"

"I guess I'm scared that Nate's going to have called the office and I wasn't there. I really love Nate. He's a good man. I don't want to hurt him, and I sure don't want to lose him. These other guys—it's just something I've done for a long time. You think this dry mouth thing means I'm scared?"

"Are you?"

"Well, Nate's so laid back and unsuspecting, I would have said I wasn't worried about it, but maybe the dry mouth thing means I really am worried, scared of losing him."

Keep in mind that there are certain types of medication that can cause a dry mouth, but for the most part, a dry mouth is a sign of nervousness or just plain fear. By honestly acknowledging your fears, if only to yourself, you may be able not only to better deal with them, but also to rid yourself of this troublesome function of the body's fight or flight response.

If you experience dry mouth frequently, it can mean that you travel much of the time in the fight or flight mode. "Why am I always so anxious?" you may ask yourself. "I hate being tense."

Perhaps, for reasons you have not examined, you don't hate it quite as much as you think. In each of the above examples, there's a common ingredient. Milton "dreaded" possible reprimands from his father and perhaps from me as a father figure. Margie "dreaded" her husband's anger. Yet in both these instances, they continued to behave in a manner calculated to place them at risk for something they said they dreaded. But in each case as well, the possibility of being taken to task for their actions by powerful figures in their lives was preferable to being ignored. Each had discerned, despite radically different situations, that negative involvement, the threat of being lectured or discovered, meant they were getting attention, and any attention was better than none at all.

If you experience a dry mouth frequently, try to discover what the payoff might be for being so consistently nervous. If you can figure it out, rather than act it out, chances are you'll be more relaxed and your dry mouth will moisten up.

THE EYES

Twitches

If, as the adage says, the eyes are the windows of the soul, then they are also good indicators of that which goes on in the psyche.

We've already discussed some of the primary responses of the body's red alert system. In the fight or flight mode, the blood is diverted to the large muscles, nonessential functions are put on hold, and adrenaline is released. Some of the other functions included in the "scrapping or scramming" mode is an increase in the clotting factors in the blood (in the event of wounds or injury) and the fact that the eyelids go on hairtrigger alert in case of an attack to the face. The eyes, of course, are essential to the defense system.

In many of the Oriental martial arts, one of the disciplines taught is the ability to fix an opponent with a baleful, unblinking stare. This is thought to be essential in gaining a psychological advantage over an opponent. The ability to stare someone down is an indicator of fearlessness.

Experiencing twitches or tics in the eye area, on the other hand, indicates the opposite. It means that you are bracing yourself for attack, that you are feeling threatened, nervous, and inadequate to the situation at hand.

Many of us—too many—have had the experience of having our faces slapped at one time or another, and the eyelid twitch can also indicate that a present circumstance is triggering a memory of some kind of former attack, whether physical or verbal.

Pamela T., a graduate student in psychology, had been raised by her grandmother, a woman who never let her forget that if it wasn't for her, she would have been in an orphans' home or worse. A harsh woman, the grandmother was hard on the little girl and left Pamela with a poor sense of self-esteem and feelings of inadequacy. Now that she was finishing up her work on her Ph.D., Pamela encountered a crusty old professor who gave her what she called "a really hard time": questioning her conclusions, the quality of her work, and her fitness for her chosen profession.

Suddenly, in midsession she blurted out, "Grandma always said I'd never amount to anything. Maybe she was right." At that confession, her eyelid began to twitch uncontrollably. Embarrassed, she covered the eye with one hand and went on talking.

"It's the same, isn't it? The way my professor and Grandma make me feel. Like they're doing me a favor just letting me stay. That's how he made me feel today. Like I really wasn't bright enough to be in the department at all and that I was only there because he felt sorry for me."

"Have you always had the twitchy eyelid?" I asked.

"I don't know—I do know that it shows up when I get nervous. It's as though I'm expecting an attack, expecting a big blowup like I used to have with my grandmother."

If you experience a twitch or tic around the eye area, run a recent inventory of your experiences and thoughts. What are you afraid of? What are you dreading? If you can identify and release that fear, chances are that the annoying tic will subside.

Itchy Eyes

The itchy eye is not an indication of a threat. Generally speaking, it means that you are experiencing the kind of emotional response to a situation that, were you not repressing the feeling, would cause you to shed tears.

Sorrow, nostalgia, and even joy can cause us to weep. When your eyes itch, it is as though tears are ready to be shed but stopped at the eyelid.

The stimulant may be a story, a movie, a snatch of music, or one of those random thoughts, those rushes of melancholy that seem to come from nowhere.

Psychiatrists and psychologists are taught from the beginning to remain detached, aloof, and emotionally uninvolved with their patients. Quiet empathy is more productive for the patient than overreactive sympathy. There are times in my own professional practice when I have marveled at my own lack of emotion at hearing yet another gut-wrenching story from one of my patients. I rush to congratulate myself on being a real professional, able to rise above ordinary human emotion in order to be able to intervene for the highest good of the patient.

Then I find myself scratching or rubbing my eyes. So much for detachment.

One final word as you search for the cause of that itchy eyelid. Remember that when you weep for others, you weep for yourself. It means that whatever you may be hearing has struck a chord of feeling within you. You respond emotionally to external stimuli because you have felt the same way at some time for some reason. Whether it is joy or sadness, once the feeling has been identified, you can then relax into it and let it go, or cherish the moment as you feel the need.

THE RUNNY NOSE

The nose is always an eloquent speaker for your body. Connected through many nerves spread profusely in a primitive network over large parts of your brain, it is capable of transmitting many kinds of emotional messages.

A frequently missed signal is a sudden runny nose, sometimes as small as a single drip, usually limited to one nostril. This is not mucus, but more like clear water, and it will taste salty, as it is actually a tear or tears.

Physically, the tears come from the lachrymal, or tear, glands at the outer corners of your eyes. There is always a small supply of tears in the eye to keep it moist, yet tears are also a physical response to an emotional reaction.

If something happens to upset you or make you sad, it may be so slight that you are not even consciously aware of it. Certainly most feelings of sadness are not profound enough to make you burst into tears, but that doesn't mean you have no reaction at all. There is in fact an increase in tear production but not enough to overflow the eye and trickle down the face, only enough to overflow into the ethmoid sinuses, producing a sudden runny nose.

Though you may be inclined to attribute a sudden runny nose to an allergy or the onset of a cold, it is more likely to be the result of a transient feeling of disappointment, sadness, or dismay.

Sandy I., a customer service representative, was in therapy for chronic fatigue. She was relating an incident at her office a few days before.

"The boss came by and asked me where Harry was. Harry's another rep. I said he wouldn't be in until the afternoon. The boss told me to tell Harry, when I saw him, to stop by his office. He said he was sending Harry to L.A. to straighten out the Perkins account.

"I just nodded and went on typing my report, but a drop of water ran off the end of my nose. I know I get to travel a lot, but I really love L.A., and I know that Perkins account as well as Harry does. I guess it really hurt my feelings when I found out the boss was sending Harry instead of me. Harry doesn't even like L.A.—he told me so."

Why bother to notice these small slights or disappointments? It's a matter of self-consolation. Never miss an opportunity to feel sorry for yourself despite what the world may have to say about it. Face it, if you don't feel sorry for yourself, who will?

The next time you find yourself with this kind of runny nose, have a small conversation with yourself. Reassure yourself that's it's all right to cry a little, even if no one else knows you're doing it. Tell yourself it felt bad, but that the hurt will heal. Get yourself a little treat to make up for the slight or disappointment, preferably inexpensive and low-calorie. Show yourself love even when others do not.

Please remember that the accumulation of small hurts, insults, and disappointments that go unrecognized and unacknowledged keep adding up in your body's computer, like interest charges on a credit card. So take the time to console yourself for the little hurts and disappointment, or share your feelings with a friend if it is something more significant. It helps to clean up the account and keep you feeling healthy and strong. The more current you keep your emotional accounts, the less interest will accumulate. That way, you can avoid your body's presenting you with a bill you aren't prepared to pay.

THE BOWELS

Growling

Borborygmi, or the audible sound of gas moving in the intestines, can occur when you least expect it. In some persons, it can be audible to the point where it is quite embarrassing. Basically caused by gas being moved about under pressure in the intestines, a noisy bowel may be an indication that you had a passing thought and wished to express it but did not. It seems most often associated with the desire to speak while in the presence of another person.

Lara L., a forty-two-year-old nurse, was in therapy to help unravel a confusing love life. She was detailing an evening with her current amour, and I sat listening quietly. All at once my intestines began to gurgle noisily. Lara paused only momentarily to point an accusing finger at my abdomen. When I said nothing, she went on with her story.

I was well aware that I wanted to ask her to come to the point, but as her therapist, it would have been counterproductive to do so. Inwardly I found myself resenting her obvious enjoyment of the retelling of her latest escapade. The adult professional was willing to be silent, but the body, like a small, willful child, expressed my desire to speak.

If you are in company, silently listening to a discourse about which you have unexpressed opinions, your intestines may growl audibly. If that happens, run a quick scan of your feelings. You may be wanting to say something but perhaps may not even be aware of your silent wish until you hear the borborygmi. You may speak up or remain silent, but the very sound may alert you to your own desires and increase your inner awareness of your feelings.

Diarrhea

Diarrhea, or a sudden single episode of watery bowel movement, may be a message from your intestines that you are feeling aggressive or angry.

Mabel L., a forty-seven-year-old chemical engineer, came into therapy because she wanted simply to get along with others better. In one session, she recounted an incident with an associate, Toni, at work.

"Toni had invited me out to eat with her and another woman, Sally. I agreed, and as we were walking down to the restroom she said, 'Mabel, will you at least try not to hurt Sally's feelings today?' You could have knocked me flat with your little finger. I just stared at her. 'What do you mean?' I asked. 'I've never hurt Sally's feelings in my life!'

"Toni just looked at me and told me that the last time I'd gone out with them, I'd told Sally she needed to watch what she ate and cut down on her carbohydrates. She said, 'I know you didn't mean to hurt her feelings, but her boyfriend had told her she needed to lose weight the day before, and she was kind of sensitive about it.'

"I was speechless," Mabel went on. "By the time we got to the restroom, I practically made a dive for the john. At first, I didn't even know what it was, just thought it was that extra cup of coffee or something, but then I realized—I was mad. Really mad."

Many of my patients have told me that diarrhea follows or accompanies feelings of strong, sudden anger or aggression. Such episodes usually occur once, with no aftersymptoms. Without putting too fine a point on things, the message from the body here is obvious.

Chronic diarrhea, which progresses to severe colitis with bloody stools and dehydration, is seen most often in people who are externally pleasant, but are frequently full of long-term covert anger. Without therapy, these patients are frequently treated with drastic surgery, and sometimes even then, continue to have symptoms.

Constipation

Constipation, or the inability to have regular bowel movements, is a traditional concern of older people and young mothers. The problem affects far more women than men, and it usually occurs on an intermittent basis. Even with today's emphasis on healthier, high-fiber diets, the problem of irregularity continues at least occasionally to affect a large segment of the population.

Chances are, as a child, you were taught to feel proud of a bowel movement and associate the passing of fecal waste with a sense of accomplishment. As young childhood and toilet training passed, however, bowel movements more than likely became associated in your subconscious with "the letting out" of equally unpleasant words and feelings. It doesn't take a child very long to realize that the accomplishment of a bowel movement is of no special importance to the world at large and that in fact the event is better kept to ourselves.

We learned at the same time that "nasty" feelings and words are also best kept to ourselves. Unpleasantness in all forms was something best kept quiet.

It is no accident that constipation affects more women than men simply because women are, traditionally at least, taught not to assert themselves in the face of aggressive, troublesome, difficult, or obnoxious people and situations.

But man or woman, chances are if you find yourself holding back feelings of sadness, resentment, or anger, you will find yourself holding back other unpleasantness, like feces, as well. Constipation can almost always be seen as a body signal of people who are inclined to "suffer in silence" and withhold their opinions for fear of displeasing others.

Shirley L., a thirty-one-year-old bank teller, was a member of one of our psychotherapy groups. She was consistently quiet and agreeable, keeping a discreet, noncommittal silence most of the time. During one of the meetings, however, she remarked that she was having trouble with constipation.

"I wouldn't bring it up, because it's pretty embarrassing, but you always say that if something is bothering you, it helps to talk about it. I've tried everything; nothing seems to help. I'm getting kind of desperate." She looked hopefully around the room, her face asking for help.

One of the more forthright and blunt-spoken members of the group answered slowly, trying to curb her natural brusqueness. "Well," she said, "if you spoke up a little more, let some of your real feelings out, you might be able to let some of your shit out, too." There was a general murmur of assent from the rest of the group.

Shirley flushed, remained silent, and looked at the floor.

The next week in our individual session, Shirley began to talk about growing up as a middle child, caught between a dominant older sister and an aggressive younger brother. She'd always had trouble holding her own, she confided, and her parents did little to intervene in the siblings' squabbles. It didn't take her long to learn that if she kept her feelings to herself, she could avoid confrontations. She'd kept up this mode of behavior well into her adult life, pushed into the shadows by the demands of a self-indulgent husband and aggressive children.

It became apparent during the course of Shirley's therapy that if she was placed under stress, she held her feelings back and her problem with constipation grew worse. Once she was able to identify the circumstances that had placed her under stress and was able to discuss her feelings freely, the constipation abated and normal bowel movements returned. Other members of the group continued to encourage her to speak up, and in private session, we continued to explore the reasons why she hesitated to do so. Gradually, Shirley learned to express herself without fear of confrontation or recrimination, and her problems with chronic constipation lessened.

If you are troubled by this problem, try to be more aware of why you are holding in your opinions as well as your bowel movements. As you begin to feel more courageous, volunteer those ideas and opinions even when you think they might meet with some disapproval or offense. Experiment a bit with being unpleasant or even downright disagreeable. Bowel movements themselves can be unpleasant and disagreeable, but they are essential to good health. When you begin to recognize the necessity of letting out unpleasantness, whether physical or emotional, chances are your problems with irregularity will subside.

HEMORRHOIDS

A hemorrhoid is a small rupture in one of the veins around the anus. Usually about the size of a pea, hemorrhoids result when blood concentrates in a weakness in the vein wall, swells, and becomes itchy or painful.

Ordinarily when the anal muscles are relaxed, the blood moves through the anus to rejoin the network of veins in the abdomen, pumping blood upward toward and through the heart. Ideally, the anal sphincter muscles are relaxed enough to allow blood to circulate through the anus but tight enough to keep feces in the rectum until the next bowel movement.

When you are excessively nervous, however, the anal muscles tighten up to the point where circulation is interfered with, squeezing the circulating blood backward. The blood then collects in a vein, and it swells up or causes a rupture in the vein wall and remains outside the rectum. Hemorrhoids can be quite painful and are usually the result of a combination of standing up for too long a time, excessive tension, and squeezing the anal muscles.

I encountered this unpleasant and painful body signal when I had just finished my internship. At last a "real doctor," a full-fledged licensed physician, I was accepted on the staff of our local hospital. To show my gratitude, I volunteered to work the emergency room on the Fourth of July. My first call came as I sat down to breakfast, and I went roaring off to practice what I'd been training for these past ten years. I never went home that day as the cases marched through—vomiting, sprained ankles, fractured toes, poison ivy, and migraine headaches. I swabbed, sutured, gave injections, wrapped casts, and prescribed medication after medication. In retrospect, I realize that it was also the first time I had no one's medical opinion to rely on but my own. No more senior resident or more experienced physician—and no room for second guesses. Relaxing was out of the question.

It was two o'clock in the morning before I staggered home, tired but giddy with the awareness that I had just experienced my first full day of what I would be doing for the rest of my life. I sank gratefully into the nearest chair and bolted out of it when I became aware of a feeling very close to what it must be like when a wasp crawls into your underwear! It was a memorable experience.

To become more aware of what happens preceding the formation of a hemorrhoid, tighten up the muscles around your anus, maintain that tightness for several hours, and walk around a lot during that period. Before you know it, you will have formed a hemorrhoid. If you happen to be pregnant, it will happen a lot faster.

On the other hand, if you don't want to get hemorrhoids or if you know from experience that they're worth avoiding, learn to pay some attention to your anal area. At the first sign of irritation, be alert to the tension that you've been carrying around, and find a way to relax. Many sufferers have found the simple exercise that follows to be helpful.

Unlock your knees, and bend them slightly. Reach back and pat your own buttocks to make sure they feel loose, first the left, then the right. Concentrate on relaxing until you're quite sure the anal area has loosened up sufficiently to restore normal circulation. It's a simple maneuver, but it works!

The emotional dynamics of hemorrhoid formation and constipation are similar, and it is not mere coincidence that these conditions sometimes occur together. But if you can find some way to slip away from your tensions for just a moment or two and loosen up, it will be worth it to your mind and your body.

THE YAWN

The yawn is a widely recognized and accepted signal from the body. It is usually interpreted as boredom or fatigue.

Scrutinized more closely, however, the yawn can be translated more specifically. Because the yawn is a prelude to sleep, and sleep is a refuge from unhappy situations or moods, the yawn can then be translated as the body's response to something you want to escape or get away from, in short, something that you don't like at all.

For example, American soldiers were amazed at the response of Viet Cong soldiers who, when captured, were bound hand and foot and dumped unceremoniously on the ground outside interrogation centers to await their turn for questioning. Fully aware of the brutal methods used by the Vietnam interrogators to elicit information from captive soldiers, they did not await their turns in alert or cringing apprehension. Instead, they fell asleep.

The value of sleep as an escape is not unfamiliar to any of us, and the yawn as the harbinger of sleep is a clear indication that something is happening that is making you yearn to escape the circumstance through sleep.

Alex G., a forty-eight-year-old claims adjuster, told of meeting his future son-in-law for the first time. "It was early in the evening, and I wasn't at all tired, but as soon as we'd started to talk, I had to stifle a yawn. It was embarrassing."

"Were you bored?"

"Not at all. He's a very interesting young man. He's been all over Europe on business, speaks fluent German and Spanish, and was very well mannered. But I just couldn't stop yawning.

"I finally lied and said I'd gotten up unusually early that morning. But I knew I wasn't sleepy, and I wasn't bored. What was going on?"

"How did you feel about him?"

"I like him, I guess. He certainly doesn't beat around the bush about anything. And my daughter is certainly taken with him. She hangs on his every word, like she's hypnotized or something."

"You mean she hangs on his every word the way she used to hang on yours?"

"Maybe," Alex agreed reluctantly and yawned elaborately.

"And perhaps you found the young man more irritating than you're willing to admit?"

"He was pretty self-confident for somebody meeting his fiancée's parents for the first time," Alex admitted grudgingly. "I guess I was put off by the fact that he treated me not like a future father-in-law, but more like, well, like an equal. I mean, he may be a Washington big shot, but to me, he's still just some kid trying to take my daughter away from me. There. I've said it. I feel stupid, but I said it."

"And your yawn said it first," I reminded him.

Linda T., a thirty-nine-year-old computer programmer, was worried about her teenage daughter's behavior. "She lies all the time, says she's going to spend the night with a girlfriend and when I check up on her, she isn't there.

"Take the other night. I was going to spend the night with my boyfriend, and at sixteen, she's old enough to stay by herself. I had to tell her I was going out of town, because I know how she resents it when I spend time with Mark. She said it was fine with her to stay by herself, and we set the rules. No parties, that kind of stuff. But around midnight, I don't know, I got worried about her, so I hopped in the car and drove by the house. There was this friend's of hers—a boyfriend's—car in the driveway. I was furious! You can't trust her."

"Why do you think she lies?" I asked her.

Linda stifled a huge yawn. "I don't know. I've always

taught her to tell the truth, to be up front with me." She yawned again. "Are you saying it's my fault she doesn't tell the truth?"

"Am I bringing up something you don't want to discuss?"

"I swear, you psychiatrists are all alike. Whatever happens to a child is automatically the mother's fault. Never mind that her father ran out on us. I'm sick of it. I come here for help and all I get are accusations."

I proceeded cautiously. "I guess I was wondering if maybe the reason she thinks it's all right to lie to you is because she knows you sometimes lie to her."

Linda frowned. "Okay, you've made your point. I do lie to her sometimes." Once again, Linda yawned. "I hate listening to this kind of stuff."

So watch that yawn. It can be telling you there's something going on, whether externally or internally, that you'd prefer to be away from, to escape, or to sleep through. It may be saying, "I hate this kind of stuff."

Part Two

Louder Cries from the Body

INTRODUCTION

Though the body messages in the first part of this book, the whispers, are often quiet or brief enough to be passed over or forgotten, this part concerns itself with the body's more urgent messages, signals that are much more uncomfortable and therefore much harder to ignore. Left unacknowledged or untreated, these louder messages from the body can lead to illness, sometimes serious illness. On the other hand, an increased understanding and grasp of the messages here can hasten the healing of an illness or sometimes enable you to avoid an illness altogether.

I'm aware that there are those of you who find the notion that your mind can make you sick quite without foundation. A few years ago, I would have said the same thing myself. Still the evidence of the connection between the mind and the body is there and can be seen over and over again. When that connection is acknowledged, the emotions that cause negative body events and illnesses can be expressed in other healthier ways.

I know that I make it sound easier than it sometimes is. It's one thing to know how your mind and emotions work, but it can be quite another to change your mental habits. In dealing with the body's more insistent messages, be sure to give yourself adequate time, patience, and practice. Get professional help if you need it. Those things we call neuroses and the attendant physical problems they can cause don't develop overnight; often they don't go away overnight either. But the physical signals and emotions that I've identified here will give you a place to start.

Meanwhile, always seek the help of your family physician, even though you may be trying to figure out your feelings at the same time. Do not neglect or avoid medical treatment, even if you know what emotional transaction triggered the illness.

These are potentially serious illnesses and must not be ignored.

BACK PAIN

Upper Back Pain

One of the more fascinating aspects of the body–mind connection is the body's ability to sometimes translate the emotional reactions common to us all in an almost literal way. This is particularly true in the case of the sudden and often quite debilitating type of upper back pain caused by a spasm of the muscle between the ribs and under the shoulder blades. Let's look at a couple of examples.

Freda L., a forty-two-year-old caterer, settled herself carefully in a chair in my office, obviously experiencing a great deal of pain. She explained that she experienced the onset of the spasm two nights before. It was so bad at first that both she and her husband had been sure she was having a heart attack, though the pain was located in the back and not the front of the chest wall. A trip to the emergency room and a thorough examination had led to a diagnosis of muscle spasms and a prescription for pain medication. But clearly, Freda was still suffering.

"When you feel a terrible pain like this, it can mean there's a powerful emotion going on," I told her. "Is there any new problem going on, something you're worried about?"

Freda shook her head. "I knew you'd ask me that. Nothing. At least, well, nothing. I don't know what it could be."

"How's your husband?" I persisted gently.

"Fine. He's been given some new responsibility at work, but everything seems to be going well."

"And Cathy?"

At the mention of her teenage daughter, Freda's face went ashen. "Oh, my Lord," she breathed. "I've been so preoccupied with this pain! I almost forgot about her.

My God! She's pregnant! And she told me about it the day before yesterday. Just came in cool as you please. She said she didn't want me to get excited!"

"What did you do?"

"I controlled myself as well as I could. I asked her if it was her boyfriend's baby, and she said that it was. She told me she thought they were too young to get married but that she wanted to have it anyway. She wanted to know if her father and I would help her raise it!"

Freda sighed heavily. "It was all I could do to sit there without screaming. How could she do something like that? Just expect her father and I to take on a, well, an illegitimate baby to raise. At our time of life. What will everybody think? I don't know what we're going to do. She's my only child—I had such high hopes for her, for her future. And now this."

She stared sightlessly at the floor. "I know it's old-fashioned these days, but Ben and I never did anything until we were married. I feel—I feel like she's betrayed me."

"Like she stabbed you in the back?" I offered.

Freda's eyes widened with recognition. "That's exactly what it feels like," she admitted. "Like she stabbed me in the back."

Freda's intense pain lasted for days afterward. But as she gradually adjusted to her family's crisis, it gradually abated.

My own experience with a muscle spasm of this kind also had to do with feelings for a daughter. My wife and I were on the way to a restaurant for dinner when I was seized by a stab of pain so acute that I had to pull off the road. I had to hang on to the steering wheel to keep from falling out the door.

My wife was terrified. "What is it? What's wrong?"

I reviewed the events of the past hour, trying to identify what it was that had hit me so hard. All at once, I knew. I sat there, feeling pretty foolish for my histrionics. The pain began to ebb away but still throbbed uncomfortably. I explained to my wife what was going on.

We'd gone through the day's mail before we left the house and among the letters was a large manila envelope from my daughter. She'd sent us a copy of her latest literary effort from one of her writing classes, and I was impressed with her masterful writing. My wife and I had discussed it briefly, returned the piece to the envelope, and headed out for dinner.

What my body knew and felt was that my daughter was not only a good writer, she was a better writer than I was! Ashamed and embarrassed, I attempted to confide my feeling of jealousy and betrayal to my wife. Here I was, making all the sacrifices to send her to college, and she turns around and stabs me in the back. It felt terrible to say it, but I had to be as honest as my body had been with me.

My wife, who has grown used to my neurotic blitherings, studied me for a long moment. "You should be glad she's good," she said after a moment. "She can make better use of a talent for writing than you can. You already have a profession."

I'd like to report that the pain in my ribs subsided after my disclosure, but that wasn't the case. We went on to the restaurant, but after dinner, it started up again. I knew I was in for a long, sleepless night. What kind of father was I to feel such competition with my own child? What kind of egocentric, selfish person could think this way?

Obviously, I could, which can only serve to bring home the point that emotions are not rational responses to our experiences. An emotional reaction can seem to be completely alien to the way you think about yourself. Yet, stupid as you might think a feeling is, an emotion can nevertheless demand your attention and examination. In my own case, the pain under my ribs did not entirely subside until I called my daughter to discuss my envy of her fine writing. She was very understanding, and at last, I got some relief.

Low Back Pain

Low back pain usually strikes where the vertebrae join the pelvis, resulting in muscle spasms in the surrounding area. It may be a problem that develops gradually, or it may strike very suddenly to get your attention. In many cases, it can develop into a chronic and debilitating condition. Much has been written about low back pain and its connection to certain psychological states, but basically, the pattern is as follows.

As with most of our emotional experiences, the body seems to translate an emotional posture into a fantasied physical experience. In this particular case, the main hinge in the backbone, between the upper and lower body, the lumbosacral joint, tightens up as though you were carrying a heavy weight on your shoulders. The muscles surrounding the joint get fatigued, then go into spasm. The strain on the muscles in turn causes more pain and fatigue as the cushions between the vertebrae are compressed. The pain reaches an intolerable level and can lead to complete incapacitation.

Why? If, in fact, the body is translating an emotional posture, then low back pain can be linked to a feeling of being overburdened, just as if the emotions had physical mass and weight. If you are going through a time in your life when you feel constantly vigilant or "on duty," always responsible, you may see yourself as weighted with responsibilities. Emotionally, you may desire rest, relaxation, and attention or acknowledgement from those around you, but you won't let yourself ask for those things or unburden yourself to others. The metaphorical weight of your responsibilities is too great. You continue to shoulder your emotional burden until your back gives you no choice but to acknowledge the strain. Incapacitated by low back pain, you are forced to lie down, feel sorry for yourself, and garner some needed care and attention from those around you.

Frequently, people who are experiencing low back pain may be in a position where they are caretaking for others and secretly wishing to lay the burden down and let someone take care of them for awhile.

Opal H., a thirty-eight-year-old dietician, was deeply concerned for her mother-in-law when she was quite unexpectedly widowed. Her mother-in-law had always been highly dependent on her husband and felt hopeless and alone after his death. Opal and her husband discussed it and, after some deliberation, invited the woman to live with them at least until she could better adjust to her situation. But Opal's mother-in-law began to be as dependent upon her son as she had once been upon her husband. Once a pleasant guest in their home, she became demanding and querulous.

As the situation worsened, Opal developed a nagging lower back pain as a result of not only her increased responsibility, but the loss of attention from her husband and the guilt she felt over the fact that when it came right down to it, the situation was untenable; she wanted her mother-in-law to move out. When the elderly woman finally did so, sharing an apartment with another widow, Opal's pain gradually abated, and things returned to normal.

In other instances, the burden may not be one of real responsibility, but an imagined or fantasized one. Frank P., a fifty-four-year-old bank manager, began a "harmless" flirtation with a young female neighbor who was fond of tanning in a rather tantalizing bikini. While his wife was out working, Frank would find all sorts of excuses for coming home in the middle of the day. He would lean on the fence and allow himself to be charmed and excited by the neighbor's friendly conversation. Frank's fantasies of a liaison with this young woman increased to the point where they actually became a kind of emotional burden, and Frank developed chronic low back pain.

On the advice of his physician, he took to his bed for several days. As he lay there, stricken, gazing out the window at his bewitching young neighbor, he realized that his half-formed plans and fantasies of a torrid affair were ruining his life. The burden of guilt those fantasies had created were too much—his back literally bent under the burden. Once he gave up his plans for an assignation, the guilt disappeared and so did his back pain.

THE NECK AND SHOULDERS

Despite their close physical proximity, pains in the neck and shoulders can be the result of very different sets of feelings.

Neck Pain

Consider the common expression: "____ is a pain in the neck." You can fill in the blank with a person, a particular situation, or task. Yet, if you physically experience a pain in the neck, your first thought is almost invariably, I must have slept wrong, not, as is more often the case, Who or what is giving me this pain in the neck?

Over years of listening and working with hundreds of people who have learned to listen and to decode their body's messages, I've found that a pain in the neck can be almost invariably traced back to feelings of irritation, displeasure, or pique, whether resulting from a real or fantasied transaction. It is as though an unpleasant emotional (psycho-) event is perceived by the body (-somatic) as an actual trauma to the neck.

Again, going back to the fight or flight response, when you receive or anticipate a psychic trauma, the muscles in the neck tense up in order to better absorb the blow or attack. Continued tension results in pain in the little muscles that run in chains up and down the cervical vertebrae on either side of the neck. Sometimes a chain on one side will contract more than the one on the other, actually pulling the neck to one side. Still more tension results in muscle fatigue and increased pain.

A chiropractor can sometimes help muscles to relax

through massage or manipulation, but more often the pain will disappear when the source of tension or displeasure is identified, acknowledged, and released. But, if left unattended, neck pain can be quite serious because the contracted muscles can squeeze to the point where they put pressure on the nerve roots of the spinal cord. In some situations, surgical intervention may be required to relieve it.

Alicia F., a thirty-four-year-old office worker, appeared at one of our sessions wearing a semisoft neck brace. When I inquired about it, asking her what had happened to give her a pain the neck, she only shrugged at first.

"I don't know," she answered. "Our family doctor took an X ray and prescribed this collar. He said if it hadn't gotten any better by next week, he'd have me go see an orthopedic surgeon. I don't know how I hurt it, though. Maybe it was sleeping in front of the air conditioner."

She moved her head slightly and winced. "All I know is that it hurts all the time."

"How long have you had it?"

"Since Saturday. My brother-in-law and his family are visiting us, and we were sitting around talking. All at once it tightened up, and it's been giving me fits ever since."

"How long are they going to stay?"

Alicia sighed audibly. "A week. And they've got these three kids. You know how kids are. Running all over the place. I mean, I know they're just kids, but when they knocked over that lamp, I could hardly control myself."

"What happened then?"

"The parents didn't seem to care very much. And I couldn't say anything because I know what they think of us. Me and George, two jobs, no kids. I guess they think we should live in a tiny apartment like they do and never have anything. I don't want to make them feel unwelcome, but those kids are tearing everything up!"

"It must be a real change for you and George to have all those kids around," I offered.

"Running up and down the stairs, climbing on the couch, carrying food all over the place!" Alicia's voice rose miserably. "If they knew how we've scrimped and saved to get that house the way we wanted it. But they just make fun of us, I know it!"

Suddenly, her face contorted and her eyes filled with tears. "They're destroying my beautiful house. My beautiful furniture! I'm afraid to go home for fear of the damage they've done while I was out. It's not fair! They don't have anything, and they don't want us to have anything either! They want those little monsters of theirs to tear up our dream house. I wish they'd go home! My house isn't ever going to be the same! I hate them!"

Her sobbing rose to a crescendo and finally slowed down again. As she dried her eyes, she was suddenly embarrassed by her outburst. "I'm sorry," she said. "I honestly had no idea how much their being here was bothering me."

"You had a lot of feelings you were holding in," I agreed. "I think they might have been giving you that terrible pain in the neck. How does it feel now?"

Cautiously, she moved her head around, her eyes wide with astonishment. "I can't believe it. It doesn't hurt anymore!"

Hastily, I cautioned her to take it easy and asked her not to expect too much all at once. I told her to keep wearing the collar as her doctor had advised and to go see him before removing it.

The next day, she telephoned to say it was almost completely well. She also said her houseguests had cut short their visit and gone home that morning.

• • •

Most of the time, the source of your sudden, sharp pain in the neck will be pretty obvious once you've formed the habit of looking for the reason for it. It is the body's way of letting you know that you just don't like something or someone at a particular moment. When you figure out what's causing it, the pain in the neck frequently disappears shortly thereafter. But do pay attention to pain or discomfort in the neck and have it checked out by a doctor if it doesn't clear up in short order. Accumulated neck pain can cause spasm, torticollis, or a squeezed intervertebral disk, and then you've got a serious problem.

Shoulder Pain

Shoulder pain is another event that can send you off to the nearest chiropractor or orthopedic surgeon. Muscle pain in the shoulders can be the result of conditions such as bursitis or arthritis, but it can never hurt to take a quick inventory of what's going on inside on the emotional level.

Mathilda R. was a fifty-one-year-old professor of English who had come into therapy because of a low-grade, chronic depression that had begun to interfere with her lectures and her writing. During our last two or three sessions, she had also begun to complain about excruciating pains in her shoulders, especially the right one.

A creative and energetic woman, she was the only female full professor at the university, a faculty so controlled by males, she told me, it was assumed that she, as the only female present at the board meetings, would keep the minutes.

"I was one of four girls and my brother, the only boy, always got the best of everything. I think my father was actually ashamed that his masculinity had not exerted itself enough to produce more than one boy among five children. Of course, they were proud of me when I got my Ph.D., but they never really expected me to do anything with it."

Mathilda confided that she was on the Search Committee for the new chair of the English department but was increasingly troubled by the fact that the dean hadn't encouraged her to apply for the position herself.

"I know I'm better qualified than most of the candidates we've interviewed. I could put up my own name and get backing from other committee members as well. But I don't know, I'd rather be asked. Can you understand that?"

"Have you seriously thought of putting up your own name?" I asked.

"Well, the idea has occurred to me, but I don't think they'll ever have a woman chair in that department, at least, not in my lifetime. And I am the first woman to ever make full professor there. I guess I can be satisfied with that much."

"Are you satisfied?"

Mathilda smiled ruefully and shrugged.

"I wonder if you don't want it more than you're willing to admit," I told her.

She was silent for a long moment. When she spoke again, it was in a low monotone. "You know, Doctor. You may be right. The thing is, I can't even let myself think about being chair. It doesn't seem right. Yet, if I'm really honest with myself, I know I want it more than anything. It's as if I'm reaching for it in spite of myself, like reaching for the Holy Grail."

"Hence the shoulder pain?" I said.

She shook her head slowly. "I don't know, that seems a little far-fetched. I'll have to think about it."

Over the following weeks, Mathilda and I continued to discuss the fact that she wanted the job. The more she talked about it, the more she expressed her longing, the less her shoulders ached.

Eventually, a new chair was chosen, and it was not Mathilda. She had been right about their just not being ready for a woman in the position. But the pain in her shoulders gradually subsided and finally disappeared.

If your shoulders and arms ache, try to get in touch with that something you want so much that your arms and shoulders quite literally ache from reaching out for it, ache to hold it. A job you don't think you'll get, an old flame you thought you were over, a raise, or a trip. What is it that you secretly want? Yearning is not just a pipe dream. It is as real an emotion as any other. If you recognize the feeling, express it to yourself and to as many others as you can. Admit that you are allowing yourself to want something desperately, more than you have ever wanted anything before. Perhaps by expressing these yearnings, you can move one step further to attaining the object of your desires.

As close as the neck and shoulders are to one another, the hidden emotions that cause discomfort in these areas can be very different indeed. If you suffer discomfort in either the neck or the shoulders, have a little talk with yourself and identify what's really going on. Is something giving you a pain in the neck? Or are you silently reaching out for your heart's desire?

SCOLIOSIS

Scoliosis is one of the more obviously psychologically caused ailments that fairly begs to be analyzed and treated psychotherapeutically. However, it is a condition that is seldom or not at all, in my experience, treated in the psychiatrist's consulting room.

At the time when the condition is remediable, that is, in childhood, the decision for or against therapy is in the hands of the parent. Even if the mother happens already to be in therapy herself, she might find it difficult, if not impossible, to believe that her young daughter (60 to 80 percent of the cases are girls) could have this crippling condition caused by something so innocuous as a desire to be shorter.

All of the children with scoliosis that I have seen were brought in by mothers who happened already to be in therapy with me. Because they were beginning to think about mind–body connections, they wondered if the child's emotions might be involved in the lateral curvature that had been first noticed during routine school physical exams.

Although their instinct was sound (I was quite sure it was psychosomatic), none of them, in my experience, was really convinced enough to go the therapy route for the children. Upon reflection, I suspect that I was not skillful enough in my efforts to bring the cause and effect to the attention of the mothers. If I had been, perhaps some of them would have opted for psychotherapy with a child psychiatrist. As it happened, in every case, the child went on to treatment with the orthopedic body braces, which cleared up the physical condition pretty well. How the emotional posture fared, we can only conjecture.

Scoliosis is a lateral curvature of the spine. Most often, it is *idiopathic*, meaning no one knows what causes it. Perhaps you and I can see a pattern here that can help to explain it.

In most people, the little stack of spools we call vertebrae, or the backbone, when viewed from the back, is straight up and down, so that the head sits directly above the tailbone, with a smooth straight row of vertebral processes running upward from the tailbone to the skull.

In the condition of scoliosis, the spine curves in an S shape left and right, with the right shoulder usually higher. Because this shift can cause pressure on nerves in the back, trouble in the hips, and even pains in the legs and neck, it must be treated by appropriate braces until it is straightened out and the pressures are relieved.

Why does it occur? Sloppy posture, say the orthopedists. Bad habits, perhaps. One leg is too long, say the chiropractors. Maybe.

An interesting circumstance is that these children are all taller than they want to be. You have only to ask them, "Would you rather be bigger or littler?" and they will almost invariably say they prefer to be littler (shorter). Usually they are charmingly open and undefended in this declaration. For a psychiatrist who deals almost exclusively with adults, it is always a pleasant surprise to deal with the innocent, un-self-conscious candor of the child.

On the other hand, if you pose this same question to the adult with scoliosis, she has long since buried her true feelings in layers of rationalizations. It may take weeks of careful layer removal to help her get in touch with the feeling of childhood: "I hated being so tall. I wanted to remain little, like I had been before."

Why do these children long for this? The answer is that children who have been petted and complimented as in "What a cute little child you are!" suddenly realize they are no longer little. Shorter is synonymous with littler, hence, younger, hence, more deserving of the attention of a doting parent.

Also, most of the time, they have younger siblings who have usurped their position in the family. It is a disturbing awareness for a young child to realize that she (or he) has grown taller and can no longer qualify for the delightful diminutive adjectives that were at the core of former parental attention. Though the child may coo to the new baby or go through the pretense of loving the new sibling in order to avoid family displeasure, it is hard to be displaced by one whose only claim to attention is its small size.

If she were aware of it and able to voice her feelings, she might cry out, "I want to be the littlest one in the family the way I used to be. Why do I have to be a big girl? I hate it. I want to be shorter and littler, so everybody loves me like they do the new baby."

But she can't say this. She would be laughed at and told she was jealous, as if that were a bad thing. So she slumps sideways and tries to be less tall. She tries to curve in on herself, and her back bends sideways.

In addition to the desire to receive the "cute little child" attention from adults, the adolescent girl realizes that most boys don't pay much attention to girls who are taller than they are. The girls who are the same height as or shorter than the boys get more flirtatious remarks and attention.

Grade school class pictures of men and women who have scoliosis frequently show them to be a half head taller than their classmates. Yes, they will admit ruefully, they were always the tallest one in the class. No, they didn't like it.

But what is a poor girl (or boy) to do? The best she can, which is to inconspicuously slump sideways and try to be short—and develop scoliosis.

Upon reflection, I wonder that I did not develop scoliosis myself, for the dynamic setup was just right. I was competitive with my younger siblings, envied their protected state, and had always, reluctantly, assumed the responsibility for their welfare. Early adolescent pictures of me show a skinny boy with one shoulder higher than the other. But some forgotten significant person complimented me in such a way that it made being tall more acceptable to me. As receptive to and hungry for praise as I was (and still am), I swelled up and stood taller and so escaped scoliosis.

THE STOMACHACHE

Molly T. was on the heavy side but attractive and well groomed. She exuded self-confidence but was nevertheless defensive about coming to see a psychiatrist. "I told my doctor the problem was in my stomach, not my head, but he said it was in both, so here I am."

She looked at me sharply, ready to take me on, then tried to soften her tone. "Well, Doctor, I'm here to be helped. Ask me anything. I'll try to answer your questions as honestly as I can."

Molly was definitely the kind of person who was used to being in control, and I wanted to make her feel as comfortable as possible. "Well, I wonder if I could get you to tell me about yourself, anything that you think will help me to know who you are."

She began by telling me that she had a "very important" job and that she was the only woman in the history of the company who had ever been given this post. She went on to describe her marriage as "very pleasant," her children as "very satisfying," and except for the ongoing problem with her stomach, her general health as "very good."

Superlatives like *very* seemed to come to Molly naturally. It seemed that ordinary amounts of anything were never quite enough. She ended her narrative by saying, "So you see Doctor, I have everything I need to make me happy."

"But your stomach doesn't seem to be happy," I reminded her.

Her face clouded. "You're right. I've read about ulcers and stomach trouble. I know they say that if you have stomach trouble, it means you're hungry—for love, I guess. But I get plenty of love from my husband, my children love me, and they like me at work. Why isn't that enough?"

"Tell me about your childhood if you can," I said.

Molly's childhood was "very happy" as she described it. The youngest of three children and the only girl, she was petted and indulged. Her mother dressed her in pretty, frilly dresses, and her father would take her with him on outings, showing her off to his friends. He called her his little princess.

I asked her what was the best time of her life.

"Why, right now, I guess. It should be. I've gotten everything I've ever wanted. I have it all. Nobody could ask for anything more."

"But these stomachaches. Your chronic hunger—your stomach is asking for more. It sounds as though it's never satisfied."

Molly frowned considering it. "You're right. I don't feel as though I have any right to want more, but sometimes I find myself saying, 'Is this all there is?' It makes me feel guilty, but sometimes I know I want something else—something more—I just don't know what it is."

In subsequent sessions, Molly gradually came to grips with the fact that the best time of her life had been that halcyon period when she was her father's "little princess." That, as she said, "was a hard act to follow."

I wish that I could report that in a few brilliant hours I was able to uncover the mystery of Molly's needs that caused her stomach to grind hungrily on itself. No amount of food of any type was satisfying, and her stomach rebelled after every feeding. In desperation, she tried avoiding spicy foods, rich foods, rough-textured foods, and acid-producing foods—all to no avail. Her hunger drove her to eat when she was not really hungry, at least not hungry for food.

It was as though, partly from genetic predisposition and partly from the plethora of attention and coddling she received from her doting parents, there was some unfillable cavity inside her always wanting more and more and more. As she said on one occasion, "It feels as though if my husband stayed home with me all day long and told me every ten minutes how much he loved me, it wouldn't be enough. I can feel how hopeless it is to try to get enough, and I know I'm never going to get that big hungry roaring hole inside me filled up. What can I do?"

The change Molly gradually made to solve her problem was that instead of uniformly presenting a facade of self-sufficiency and competence and denying the hungry-for-love child inside her body, she was able, in the privacy of the therapy situation, to acknowledge her real feelings. In her sessions, she was finally able to weep and lament the loss of that wonderful time of her life that she had been led to believe would last forever.

She endured a long period of desperation as she came to grips with the fact that she could never recapture the continuous doting environment of her childhood. The relief of pressure that came with acknowledging her internal cravings finally began to pay off, though periodically she would complain that she felt worse than at any time of her life as she transferred the expression of her hunger from her stomach to her conscious awareness.

"Sometimes I feel like I'm a big empty container, and no matter how much I put in me, it's never enough. I just can't fill myself up to the top. I already eat too much food, but if I don't put in lots of food, my stomach aches and burns. More and more I'm feeling that I can never be satisfied."

Because she was dealing with early primitive feelings that had begun at a time in her life when she simply felt without reasoning, these built-in emotions were really difficult for her to resurrect.

Yet, as she discussed them, they came awake again. She felt miserable as she realized her childhood couldn't be recaptured. As she consciously experienced the emotional pain of that loss, her stomach began to relax and allow her vocal equipment to do the expressing.

Molly was one of the lucky ones who had the persistence to stay with the hard process of working through early half-forgotten feelings, and her body quieted down.

She even learned to joke about her own cravings. She tapered off her visits and finally left therapy.

As I have indicated elsewhere, as a psychiatrist, I have had a good deal of personal therapy. Not as much as I would like sometimes, but enough to be moderately comfortable with myself most of the time. If I were entirely free of neurotic feelings, it would be more difficult for me to empathize with my patients and their more troublesome symptoms and feelings. Sometimes I feel as though I have a little of every symptom each patient brings in—hopefully, under control enough to be able to help them work out theirs. Consider the aching stomach:

One day in summer, my daughter was working on a small house she designed and was building with her own hands on a corner of the small farm where we lived and where I still have my office. She was assisted by a hired man who was a willing worker but, like her, unskilled in the building arts. I had been riding the tractor, cutting weeds, wearing only shoes and a pair of cutoff jeans. She came to me and asked me to show her and Joe how to solder pipe for the plumbing.

My plan was to have Joe do it first, with her listening and observing. She squatted down to one side to watch him and listen to my directions. All three of us were very intent as I had him clean off the inside of the copper collar, then the outside of the smaller pipe that was to be soldered into the union. He applied soldering grease (flux) to the two cleaned surfaces, the outside of the smaller pipe and the inside of the larger collar, or union. The end of the smaller pipe was then slipped into the union, and he began to play the flame of the torch over the area to be soldered. When it was smoking from the flux and seemed hot enough, I directed him to apply the end of the coil of lead solder to the pipe where it went into the union, so that as it melted from the heat of the pipe, it would be sucked into the union, sealing and soldering the pipes together.

I was very intent on Joe's technique, because this was his first experience at soldering, and I wanted to be sure they both learned how to do it effectively. My daughter, who was looking back and forth between him and me, suddenly spoke up, alarmed, "Daddy, why are you holding onto your stomach?"

Because we were at the critical juncture of the procedure, I was unaware that I had hunched forward with my right hand on my stomach area, above the belt and near the midline. Not wanting to break the spell of concentration just as I was ready to tell Joe to take away the flame and let the joint cool and harden in place, I was impatient with her interruption. I paused an instant to notice that I was indeed pushing on my stomach to quiet it down. I had not noticed the sudden cramp that had made me bend forward and press on my upper abdomen. I said impatiently, "I guess I'm pushing on it because it hurts. Now, Joe, gently, let go of it and take the flame away."

"But, Daddy, why is it hurting? What's the matter with it?" my daughter persisted, getting up and coming over to me.

Touched by her concern and relaxed now that the two pipes were successfully soldered together, I looked at her thoughtfully. Talking as I was running through my own feelings, I said, "Well, I guess it's hurting because I'm telling you how to do something, and I know that whenever I try to tell you how to do something, you get mad at me—I guess I must be afraid you'll be mad at me."

"But you're trying to help me. I couldn't be mad at you for that. I love you. How can we make your stomach stop hurting?"

I ran a quick appraisal of my stomach's feelings. The cramping was gone. I grinned at her. "I guess you already have. It stopped hurting as soon as you said that. Powerful medicine." She gave me a little hug, and I went back to the tractor, and she and Joe climbed back into the building.

When your stomach bothers you, your usual response may be to wonder what you have eaten that is not agreeing with you, but chances are your discomfort has more to do with your emotions than your eating habits.

When you feel that first twinge of cramping in your stomach area, perhaps you can ask yourself if you have been rejected or disappointed or are somehow afraid that you will be cast outside a circle of acceptance by someone whose good feelings are important to you. If you can recognize the feeling and where it's coming from, you can then transfer the anxiety of rejection or emptiness from your stomach to your conscious awareness, and your stomach can relax and start doing what it does best—helping to digest food when it comes in and sitting around comfortably, resting until the next feeding.

Finally, as I have indicated elsewhere, do not neglect persistent stomach symptoms, no matter how insightful you may become. An upset stomach can move on to becoming an ulcer, and while you are becoming acquainted with your feelings, an ulcer can be serious, even fatal, if not treated. Have your family physician check your symptoms and see that they are appropriately treated.

Meanwhile when your stomach aches, think, Why am I suddenly feeling unloved?

NAUSEA AND VOMITING

Near the end of World War II, Allied troops overran Germany and liberated from the concentration camps their starving inhabitants, more dead than alive. Their captors had fled in the face of the advancing armies, leaving the gates open and their half-dead prisoners unguarded.

The majority of the victims were too weak to do anything more than stare dully at their saviors. Nearly dead of starvation and disease, they were pitiful wrecks of what had once been healthy, well-fed men, women, and children. For months prior to the liberation of the camps, encircling armies had cut off supplies to Germany, food had become increasingly scarce, and the inhabitants of the camps got almost nothing, sentenced to slow starvation. Most were too weak to stand, their bodies emaciated to the point where bones seemed held together only by taut skin, their bellies swollen with starvation.

The husky, well-fed Allied troops expressed their concern for these shuffling skeletons by sharing boxes of K-rations, rich in nourishment, high in carbohydrates, fat, and protein.

The results of this generosity were, for the most part, disastrous. The starvelings that had existed for so long on next to nothing were unable to stomach normal food; their digestive systems had ceased to function. Most were convulsed in spasms of retching, some vomited up blood, and some even died from the shock to their wrecked digestive systems.

Finally, under the care of military doctors, the starving prisoners were gradually brought back to health with slightly enriched broths that were eventually upgraded to more nourishing foods until their digestive systems could once again handle normal food intake.

A safety function of the human stomach is its ability to forcibly contract and throw back, or vomit, its contents when the body decides that what has been taken in is unsuitable or undesirable. Sometimes this happens unexpectedly in the presence of unpleasant stimuli. But sometimes the stomach will also eject its contents in the presence of pleasant or good stimuli as well.

Each of us becomes used to the kinds of food we eat, and if we are confronted with food that is outside our normal intake, we may reject it as too rich or too exotic. In the same way, our minds and emotions become used to a certain level of success and/or pleasure. When we experience something that transcends that level, it can cause us to become restless, anxious, and—you guessed it—nauseous. The body then attempts to throw back the overstimulation and return things to the level we think of as normal.

Jennifer R., an ambitious young businesswoman, was one of my "graduate students," having been in therapy long enough to overcome her panic attacks but continuing in therapy as a means of self-discovery and expansion. I was, therefore, very surprised when she called me in the middle of the night, a note of panic in her voice.

"I can't stop vomiting," she told me. "I can't even keep a glass of water down." Hurriedly, we ruled out any possibility of a virus or food poisoning. "No," Jennifer assured me. "I know it's psychosomatic. I hate to call you like this, but I don't know what else to do. I feel like I'm going to vomit myself to pieces. But I can't think what is making me feel this way. I'm scared to death."

"What happened today? Did you get any news that might have gotten to you like this?"

"Well, no—" There was a long pause on the other end of the line. "I got the job," she whispered.

It was all I could do to keep from shouting. "You got the job? The one you've been talking about for months? The one with the travel, the perks? That's wonderful!"

"That's what the vomiting is, isn't it?" Jennifer's voice was tearful, weak with relief. "Oh, God. That's it. I think it's too rich, too good for me."

"And you're trying to throw it back up," I finished. "Never mind. Have a glass of water and go to bed. You're going to be just fine."

Jennifer's emotional system was accustomed to a certain level of prosperity. She was used to her place in the pecking order at work, and suddenly she was in a position where she would be on an equal footing with her superiors. A jump in income opened up a whole new world of options that were previously unavailable to her. It was wonderful, but it was also terrifying. The new job meant a lot of changes—and some losses as well. Maybe that inner emotional voice was saying, "Maybe it's all too much. Maybe it isn't worth it. Maybe you should not accept it—vomit it up."

Nona T., a professional woman of my acquaintance and not in therapy as far as I know, set out to form an association of men and women in her field, working for various corporations in the state. Because Nona knew these businesspeople shared common problems, she figured they might increase their effectiveness by pooling their resources. After months of work writing letters and talking on the telephone, she hired a conference room at a large hotel for the first organizational conference. After mingling in the lobby with other participants, many of whom she'd never met, the appointed time grew near and she made her way toward the conference room.

Proposal in hand, it suddenly struck her that this was the culmination of months of planning and politicking, that this was it—the moment, as it were, of truth. She vomited almost without warning, throwing up punch and cookies all over the front of her suit jacket. A kind waiter helped her out with some wet towels, and Nona, a resolute sort of person, simply took off her jacket and made her way to the podium. The meeting was a resounding success, and she was unanimously elected as the organization's first president.

While Nona's situation could easily be written off as a fairly normal response to stress, it is equally valid to examine her body's language in terms of the fact that she was about to receive some cherished recognition from her colleagues, a richer and more comprehensive recognition for her accomplishments than she had ever received before. At first, success can seem awfully rich to the emotional stomach. Sometimes you'll want to throw it back up, rejecting it for some plainer form of nourishment.

So how do you adjust to success without losing your lunch? The human body can learn to live in the desert or the frozen wastelands of the Arctic Circle, but it must learn to adapt to these extremes by degrees. So it is with the rich diet of success.

If you experience waves of nausea or vomiting in reaction to fortunate events, give yourself time to adjust to your new condition by degrees. Admit that you like it, but don't gobble it all up at once. Take it in by degrees, and discuss your good fortune with friends who will support you but who are relatively uninvolved and perhaps less likely to be jealous of you. Success will then be easier to get used to.

The next time you experience an episode of nausea or vomiting, try to figure out what it is that seems too rich for you to swallow. If you identify the success trigger that is making you vomit, try to acknowledge that whatever is going on is probably a good thing. The goodness might not always be apparent, for sometimes you may experience nausea and vomiting at news that is generally considered bad, for example, the death of a relative. But if the news makes you want to vomit, chances are there might be an aspect to the situation that you are reluctant to admit. Release of an obligation? Share of an estate? You may not want to admit the hidden benefit, but your body is more candid. It doesn't know how to lie.

THE COMMON COLD

The common cold, or upper respiratory infection, is usually attributed to becoming overheated and then cooling off too rapidly or to suffering other extremes in temperature, but this has never been scientifically proven or borne out in laboratory experiments.

The cold can also be described as contagious, and researchers have identified more than one hundred serospecific rhinovirus types. It is generally accepted that one of the strains of the coryza virus moves in and causes the illness when the individual's resistance is lowered by fatigue or stress. Colds are also seen more frequently in the midphase of the menstrual cycle, which may also be a time when women are more subject to stress.

Emotionally, the process of "catching a cold" seems to go like this. The person sustains a disappointment or other cause for unhappiness, which may go unnoticed. The resistance is lowered, and one of the many strains of virus that cause the common cold infect the nasopharynx and *voila!*—a cold.

If you are in the habit of being aware of your emotions, you may notice that colds are almost always caused by feelings of unhappiness or sadness. Sometimes, those emotions are completely unacknowledged until the cold is in full swing, thereby allowing the victim to admit the feelings themselves. "I feel awful," they complain, "because I have this cold."

People in psychotherapy often notice that after they have been in the process for a period of time they don't catch as many colds. As they become more aware of their feelings, those feelings get noticed, expressed, and acknowledged before the body's resistance has been lowered.

Circumstances that may precipitate a person's catching a cold include disappointment, disparagement, rejection or ingratitude, or feeling unappreciated. Some others are dread of returning to an unpleasant situation from which you have been absent, such as the well-documented preponderance of "Monday morning colds"; unrecognized envy; or an unacknowledged feeling of guilt or fear. Even vicarious participation in a loved one's unhappiness can result in your catching a cold.

But although some come down with their colds on Monday mornings, enabling them to avoid a dreaded job, others catch their cold on or around the time of a long-awaited vacation. Coincidence? Maybe not.

Consider Arlene Z., a twenty-nine-year-old mother of three who ran her own business. A driven powerhouse, Arlene had originally come into therapy because she was having trouble slowing down and relaxing.

"When Jim and I do manage to get away for a few days, we leave the children with Mom. But I can't help myself. I worry about them all the time we're gone. I think there's this part of me that thinks I'm supposed to work all the time, and when I do finally get a chance at a vacation, I feel guilty and uncomfortable. It's as though I think I have to pay for any fun I have. So most of the time, when we get away for a vacation, I get a cold and it spoils the whole holiday.

"For a while we tried planning weeks in advance. That way, I'd usually get the cold ahead of time. But I still got colds.

"This last time was really great. I didn't get a cold ahead of time, and I didn't get one during the trip. But we've been back four days, and I've got the worst darned cold I've had in years. I'm still paying for the fun.

"You see, Mom and Dad always worked hard and encouraged us kids to do the same. They weren't mean about it, but it was pretty clear that we were expected to accomplish things. When other kids were lying around watching television, we were selling Girl Scout cookies or cleaning out the basement. I guess when I'm lying out on the beach, I still think someone is not going to approve of me.

"Now that I think about it, whenever any of us kids got sick, Mom was always really good to us. You know— soup, juice, watching TV in the middle of the day. I guess I feel if I have a cold that not only will Mom not be mad at me for not doing any work, she'll love me more and fuss over me, too." Arlene stopped, blew her nose, and stared morosely at the ceiling. "I've sure got the mother of all colds right now."

Whether your colds come on as a result of dread, unhappiness, discouragement, or disappointment, whether they are a result of guilt or fear, the emotional bottom line for cold sufferers seems to be a feeling of being unloved. Colds say, "I want someone to take care of me, I want to feel loved and protected again."

If you can recognize this feeling inside yourself and admit it, if you can allow yourself to feel sorry for yourself and find a way to give you the extra attention you crave, the body will not need to express those feelings with a cold.

The foregoing is not meant to be touted as a cure for the common cold once it has begun, but it does seem to be very helpful in preventing these episodes before they start.

THE SORE THROAT

The back of the throat (the pharynx) is in a uniquely vulnerable spot to catch germs. It is the Ellis Island of the body, the landing place for an amazing variety of incoming foreign bodies. Germs are everywhere around us, and with every breath, they are pulled into the body, bouncing off the back of the throat before the air is taken into our lungs. Please test this as you read by taking a breath with mouth closed or open, and feel the air being deflected downward off the back of your throat.

Thus, the mucus-coated surface of the pharynx is usually one of our safety barriers to fight infection, because most of the incoming germs are stuck in the mucus that coats the pharynx, running on down into the stomach, where the germs are then bathed in hydrochloric acid. Result, no infection. About a quart of this mucus runs down into the stomach every twenty-four hours, killing a lot of germs. The ones that do escape the mucus stream are usually picked up by our protective killer cells, and so the germs cause us no trouble.

Under certain conditions, however, the mucus that coats the back of the throat dries up, our natural resistance to germs dies down, and germs attack the pharynx, resulting in a sore throat. We feel the pain along with the toxic effects of the infection as it spreads to the nasal passages, the sinuses, and eventually to the rest of the body. How and why does this happen?

The ever-vigilant scorekeeper, the body, does not forget. If, for example, we are slighted, insulted, or discouraged in some way, we may not acknowledge the feeling, but the body always will. If the latest wound of the spirit we have suffered is one of several in a series, we might begin to feel sad, unloved, or unappreciated.

But the body can remember when it felt loved, and it will begin to resurrect those primitive yearnings. No matter how self-centered and unlovable we might have been when we were very young, we had only to cry out, and someone, usually Mother, magically appeared and made us feel good again.

She was always there when we needed her. If we were sad, hungry, or lonely, we cried out, and she was there. Her warm hands picked us up and held us to her breast. The built-in suction pump in the back of our throat would begin to work, and the milk would come into our throats. No matter how grievous the sadness, all was immediately right and good. The suction pump would close off the intake of air, and the muscles of the throat would contract to suck in milk. We swallowed a mouthful, then let in a breath of air. The pattern was as much a part of us as our heartbeat and may even have started in the womb.

Air in, air out. Close off air and suck in milk. The muscles of the back of the throat contracted, then relaxed, contracted, then relaxed, and so on until there was enough love and milk inside.

Minds can mature, but when we are hurt and discouraged, our feelings return to that primitive state that in times past never failed to make us feel good. The body always remains a primitive machine. Chidings, slights, rejections, and disappointments are always perceived as injuries to the spirit, and the body responds in a uniquely instinctive way with primitive emotions: pain, hunger, loneliness, fear. Only love can heal these painful feelings.

In the primitive vocabulary of the body, love is closeness, warmth, concern, and food. And when we are in the throes of primitive feelings, we yearn for that solace.

The throat contracts as though to pump in milk. It does this quietly in small unnoticed motions, and it doesn't do any good. There is no mother, no breast, no milk. The pharynx gets tired and discouraged. The mucus dries up, and local resistance weakens. We continue to breathe, and germs continue to come in and land on the unprotected pharynx. Gleefully the germs and viruses embed themselves in the vulnerable tissue, attacking and multiplying. Their toxins spread through the body.

It was probably because we were feeling sad and unloved that we became ill. The body "thinks" maybe somebody will care and come to our rescue, tenderly nursing us back to health. And we will feel loved again. Without making an audible sound, the whole body cries out, "I'm sick! Help me! Please, somebody notice me and show you care about me (the way Mother used to show it)."

What to do? How can you avoid getting ill? In this instance, how do you avoid the sore throat? The crucial step in the whole process of avoiding illness is to notice when you are hurt and to acknowledge it to yourself. If you are in touch with your body and your feelings, you will notice the insult and admit that it hurt.

If it was minor, you can safely shrug it off. If it was major, say to yourself, "Ow! That hurt!" That way, you are conscious of the feeling, and it doesn't have to be hidden in your body.

If the slight, insult, or remark was something more serious and really hurt, release the emotion from your body and mind by telling somebody or several people about it. "I didn't get the raise. Darn. I'm really disappointed." The more people you tell, the more you spread the burden around and the less the burden of pain you have to carry alone.

When I have had a discouraging day, my first inkling that something isn't right is usually as I leave the office. If I haven't admitted to myself that I've had a bad day, my throat always hurts. My next thought is usually that I'm getting a sore throat and I'm going to be sick tomorrow.

On the way home, I make an effort to run back over the day's events to see what happened that hurt my feelings. Oh, yes, I remember. John G. didn't return my greeting, as though he didn't hear me, when I passed him in the hall. And when I made that motion in the committee, nobody seconded it. And Ted didn't call me back about the tennis date. None of that stuff was major, but it all makes me feel a little down in the dumps.

That night as I lie down, I think, How will I feel in the morning? Will I really be sick? Will my wife fuss around me and give me aspirin?

In the morning, when the alarm goes off, my first thought is, Am I sick? Did my throat get worse during the night? I swallow experimentally, and there's no pain. I must confess, sometimes I'm half disappointed. I don't get to be sick and be waited on because I ran the inventory and admitted to myself I felt unloved. My sore feelings and sore throat got well during the night.

To avoid the sore throat, or pharyngitis, at the first twinge of pain, try to discover your feeling of unhappiness. Figure out why you are sad or unhappy. Admit it if you are. Feel sorry for yourself. If it's bad enough, share it with someone. When you wake up in the morning, you may have the happy experience of not having a sore throat. And if you're a little disappointed that you don't get the day off, well, admit that, too, and give yourself an extra little hug.

HEADACHES AND MIGRAINES

Volumes have been written about the causes and treatment of headaches. They can be classified as due to tension, allergies, toxins, tumors, sinusitis, hypertension, and others. Nevertheless it seems likely that they are most often due to unexpressed negative feelings of unhappiness or outrage. What is important to acknowledge about headaches is that they are not just bolts from the blue. They are caused. If we understand what is going on inside us, hopefully they can be cured.

The headache can be as transient as a momentary discomfort or so monumental, so excruciating, that you can understand the desperate act of suicide. Physically, headaches are thought to be caused by either the expansion and increased circulation of blood to the brain or by the opposite: contraction of the blood vessels, resulting in sharply decreased circulation. In my experience, however, some circumstance or some person is making the headache victim unhappy and the victim either does not recognize the emotional discomfort or is for some reason unable or unwilling to acknowledge it to herself.

Migraine headaches are an especially severe type of headache that are accompanied by a premonitory aura, disturbances of vision, gastroenteric upset, and sometimes by neurological signs that seem to result from intracranial pressures. Most migraines seem to defy successful treatment, and most sufferers carry a unique burden of intense pain and incapacitation.

In my practice, clients do not apply for treatment of physical ailments, yet I am pleased to report that sometimes after they are in therapy for varying lengths of time, they will mention that they no longer have trouble with various physical ailments and syndromes, including migraine headaches. In several of my cases where migraines had been a problem, patients spontaneously reported an abatement or remission of their headache symptoms. It is probably just as well that I was not previously aware of their problems with migraines. As much as I believe in the body–mind connection, even I would have felt intimidated at the prospect of trying to treat such a daunting disorder. I do not presume to claim that I can cure migraine headaches; I am only reporting this serendipitous finding. They get into therapy, and migraines get lost along the way.

Diane N., a fifty-three-year old librarian, told me what it was like to experience migraines. "When I have one, I'd almost rather be dead. I feel as if a cannonball has been shot into the side of my head and that it's going to explode at any moment. Most of the time, I wish it would. The pain is so intense, I can't stand to have anyone around me and I don't want to hear a sound. I want to be alone, with all the lights out and the curtains drawn. When people walk around the house, it sounds so loud, like a herd of elephants. It's horrible. My mother had them, too. She always used to say she was glad I got her brown eyes and red hair, but she was sorry I got her migraines."

Diane's natural habitat was the library where she worked. She reveled in the tranquility and peace of the stacks. At times she dreaded going home to the pandemonium of a gregarious husband and the frequent visits of her grown children and grandchildren.

"I love them to death [an interesting comment], but they certainly are full of energy, running in and out—there's always a lot of commotion. And my husband is always inviting the neighbors over, too, 'just to fill the house up' he says. 'The more the merrier.' Honestly, sometimes I think I should have been a nun so I could live in a cloister."

Diane's initial reason for coming to therapy was for help with periodic anxiety attacks. A patient, uncomplaining woman, it had never occurred to her to give voice to her true feelings about crowds and confusion. Rather, she had always considered it a flaw in her character. Instead, she tried to put on a happy, welcoming face to visitors in her household.

Yet, as she became more adept at expressing her honest feelings, she gradually began to voice her mild objections to the uproar her husband seemed to prefer. The crowds did not diminish in numbers, volume, or noise, but Diane felt freer about voicing her true feelings. And her migraine headaches eventually diminished in frequency and severity.

Her children even began to accept the fact that "Mother doesn't like bunches of people around, but if we don't crowd her, she gets along okay."

As Diane allowed herself to recognize the fact that uproar was unpleasant to her and allowed herself to voice that mild displeasure, she began to feel better. Even though her history indicated what might have been a genetic predisposition to migraines, she succeeded in lessening their intensity and severity.

Thus, headaches, if viewed as a signal, can capture your attention like a skyrocket going off. But if you can put the pain aside for a moment, ask yourself the questions: "What is going on in fact or in fantasy that I don't like? What am I objecting to?" If you can answer these questions, perhaps you can banish headaches from your life. Being able to admit that you hate something, or at least that you really dislike it, can free you from all sorts of troublesome symptoms.

Please do not expect it to be a simple task even though I have described these "cures" rather glibly. It takes a lot of work and time as well to recognize your true feelings. But if you are willing to work at it, the loss of headaches will be a special bonus.

SKIN DISORDERS

A dermatologist friend once said to me, "If the eyes are the windows of the soul, the skin is the canvas of the psyche." Indeed, my friend was aware that many of the skin disorders he treated were in fact outward reflections of inner emotional conditions.

As we discussed in the chapter on blushing, the skin will flush or blanch in response to the level of comfort or discomfort that a person is experiencing at a given moment. If that feeling lasts for more than a few seconds, the skin can begin to undergo changes that reflect that condition, ranging from the relatively slight—an itch, for example—to quite severe—eczema or other lesions.

The skin can be thought of as one of the silent communication organs of the body, projecting the thoughts and feelings of the person inside. The skin can say "I want you to like me, I want to be touched," as in the case of a sudden itch, or "I'm in conflict, I'm afraid," as in adolescent acne. When a skin condition or disorder is localized, the skin is further specifying its message to the world and, hopefully, the person who lives inside that skin as well.

Normally, the process of puberty, the transition from child to adult, proceeds in a more or less orderly fashion physiologically. As the hormonal glands begin to mature, oil is secreted onto the surface of the skin through small tubular-shaped glands to make it smooth and appealing. However, if the young man (or woman) feels conflict, fear, or ambivalence about the changes going on in his body and mind, the skin will show that conflict. The pores get blocked, the muscles surrounding them squeezing tight as the subconscious tries to "block" the change. The oil glands continue to secrete in response to increased attention to matters sexual, and before long, acne is in full swing, reflecting the inner turmoil of the individual, the excitement and anxiety apparent for all the world to see.

Sometimes the anxiety or conflict over becoming an adult will be deferred until the individual is in some irrevocably committed state of being, as in the case of acne during pregnancy, where it is clear to all the world that adulthood has arrived. The woman experiences conflicts and ambivalence about the impending change in her status. Usually the acne subsides after the baby is born. On the other hand, a teenage pregnancy can clear up a prior problem with acne. The message from the subconscious then seems to be "There, I'm doing it. I'm an adult. What a relief!"

The more comfortably you and your children can talk about growing up, the less conflict they may experience. If you are not comfortable, it might be a good idea to refer them to a therapist or give them other access to an adult with whom they can discuss things, who is not a parental or authority figure. I have many times treated young teenagers who having had the opportunity to voice their conflicts and have them addressed found their "zits" were no longer a problem.

As a psychiatrist, I have never attempted to treat or cure a skin condition, always referring my patients who were afflicted with eruptions, inflammation, or thickening of the skin to a dermatologist. Nevertheless, I can testify to the fact that as their serenity increased, their dermatitis decreased. I'd like to say it was in response to therapy alone, but usually it was a combination of therapy, a change in living conditions, or a reduction of other stress factors in their lives that resulted in the change in their skin conditions.

Sometimes the change required was quite drastic. In one case, the skin condition was cured, but the patient, alas, was lost. I had been seeing Ron C., a fifty-two-year-old insurance agent, for anxiety attacks. At my request, his wife attended one of our sessions. Although it was summertime, she wore rather old-fashioned white cotton gloves. She explained that she wore them all the time. She had chronic eczema and appeared to be allergic to a wide variety of things. The skin condition had gone on for years and was apparently incurable. During the session, it came out that her mother had lived with the couple all their married life.

Some months later, Ron's wife suffered a stroke and was kept in the hospital for several weeks, her life hanging in the balance, unconscious and on life support. Despite his grief and anxiety, Ron did confide that his wife's hands had entirely cleared. When her mind was freed of turmoil, the skin did not have to display her inner conflict. Unfortunately, she did not regain consciousness and her life support was discontinued.

Another patient, Marvin W., a thirty-five-year-old accountant, reported that his dermatologist told him that the painful redness, swelling, and peeling in his hand was possibly due to an allergy.

"But I don't get why it would only come out on my left hand. I'm right-handed."

"Is there something you do with your left hand that you don't do with your right?" I inquired.

He was silent for a few minutes, and finally, blushing, he said, "I guess I can tell you this. My wife and I haven't had sex since her hysterectomy. She hasn't seemed to want to, and I haven't pushed it." He paused and took a long breath. "Well, I have been masturbating. With my left hand, as a matter of fact. I don't know why I use that one and not the right. I guess because I was taught that it was wrong, you know. God, do you suppose that's the cause of my allergy?"

We discussed it a bit further, and by his next session, Marvin held up his left hand triumphantly. The palm was pink and clear. It seemed as though once he had voiced his conflict over masturbation out loud, his hand no longer had to express his conflict for him.

If you are troubled by a skin condition, try to understand what your skin might be trying to tell you. "Talk" to your skin in that area, examine what the connection between your emotions and your skin in that area might be. If you make the right connection and can express your feeling or conflict verbally or in some other way, chances are your skin won't have to do it for you.

PATCHY BALDNESS

Patchy baldness is not to be confused with hereditary pattern baldness, which is seen mostly in males.

The patients I have seen with scattered patchy baldness, or alopecia areata, frequently had the condition for months before they mentioned it to me. I was unaware of their problem because their wigs were generally quite indistinguishable from their natural hair. Again, I am pleased to report that many times this problem, along with so many other physical symptoms, cleared up in the course of their therapy without my being directly aware or trying specifically to treat their physical symptoms.

Even though all of these patients with alopecia had come to see me for other reasons, most of them seemed to realize the baldness was associated with "nerves." On several occasions, I remained unaware that they were bothered by alopecia until they came in wearing a new hairstyle (i.e., minus the wig) and showed me proudly that their hair was growing back in again.

The diagnosis of alopecia areata is made by a dermatologist after examining the root of a pulled hair, which has a characteristic exclamation-point-type appearance. Serum antibodies to certain body hormones may also be present. As with any body condition whose cause is unknown, stress or emotional conflicts are sometimes suspected, but the patient is usually told simply that the cause is unknown.

Dermatologists have been encouraging of the women with the disease who are forming support groups. These groups seem to concentrate on acceptance of their condition, finding the best kinds of wigs and sharing the hope that the condition might spontaneously terminate and their hair would begin to grow again. This, of course, does occasionally happen.

The support groups seem resistant to suggestions of

therapy, preferring to believe that their condition is due to some inborn error of metabolism and not due to any "nervous" ailment. However, it seems easier for women in therapy to accept that the loss of hair is a symptom of their internal anguish. Happily enough, several of my patients have been able to resolve their conflicts in psychotherapy and were delighted to find that the baldness process was arrested and, in some cases, reversed.

The precise psychological pathway for this ailment is obscure. It is tempting to speculate that in their turmoil the patients are at their wits' end and feel like pulling out their hair in frustration. Their bodies then seem to cooperate by having the smooth muscle go into spasm around the opening of the hair follicles, "strangling" the hair and causing it to fall out. Suffice it to say that many of my patients with the disorder were having conflicts and that their patchy baldness reversed and hair growth resumed once they turned the corner of their feelings and began to feel more comfortable with themselves and more conflict-free.

Elinor G. was a thirty-nine-year-old secretary who had one nineteen-year-old son. Edgar seemed always to be in trouble. During his high school years, he argued with his teachers, and when he graduated, he had trouble with his employers. His mother and father divorced when he was twelve, and he had elected to stay with his mother, although he spent days and weeks with his father, who had remarried.

As Elinor understood it, Edgar felt aggrieved that his father had left his mother for another woman but at times blamed his mother for his father's leaving anyway. He felt that life had given him a dirty deal and was angry at the world in general, and his mother in particular, for the cruel blow of losing his two-parent household.

Elinor, for her part, also took on some, if not most, of the blame for the breakup and tried to "make it up" to Edgar by being "extra understanding" in his disputes with authority figures. She was inconsistent and vacillating in trying to play the role of both father and mother. Unable to enforce any rules with Edgar, she became frightened when he began to drink beer and run with a loose crowd of boys and girls. She feared he would contract AIDS or get a girl pregnant.

Most of her sessions revolved around Edgar. I tried to encourage her to think about herself, but her guilt about not providing a stable home life for Edgar drove any consideration of her own needs from her mind.

One day she remarked that she had been to see a dermatologist about her loss of hair and leaned forward to show me the patchy white areas of baldness over her scalp. "I know it's because I worry so much about Edgar, but what can I do? He doesn't have a father, really. His dad gives him money, and his stepmother tolerates him pretty well, but neither one of them pays any more attention to him than they have to. He gets mad at me and tells me he's moving in with his father, stays two or three days, and comes home again. I have trouble concentrating on my job, too. Yesterday I forgot to remind my boss about an appointment he had, and he had to go rushing off, late. I think sometimes I'm going crazy."

"Maybe you need to worry a little more about Elinor and a little less about Edgar," I suggested gently.

"How can I? He is my child, and I know I spoil him, but the poor little guy doesn't have a whole family. I know it's really not my fault, but it is my responsibility. I don't know what to do."

"Perhaps if you hand him some of the responsibility for his own life, he might feel better about himself," I suggested, thinking that she did, indeed, have a hard row to hoe. "It seems that Edgar has been treated like a child who is unable to handle any of his own problems for so long that he thinks only you can make his life work okay. You may want to think about approaching him with the idea that you don't know how to make his life right. Perhaps you can ask him if he has any ideas about how to have a more comfortable and successful life. Hand his problem to him, or at least, let him pick up his end of the load. It would certainly lighten your burden."

Over the next few weeks, Elinor began to formulate a plan to discuss with Edgar her sense of frustration and admit that she needed his help in making things work out better. One day she reported breathlessly that they had had a long, serious talk and that Edgar seemed at first resentful but, finally, somewhat more excited and interested in undertaking the search for his own "salvation."

"That's what he said, Doctor, 'I have to find my own salvation.' He sounded more mature than ever before. I don't know if anything will come of it, but I feel like a load has been lifted off me."

Elinor and Edgar's story had ups and downs, but gradually, it began to look as though things had turned a corner. Edgar still ran with the same friends, drank beer, and had relationships with "crazy, irresponsible girls," but his mother reported with wonder that he was getting up in the mornings without her having to coax and cajole him and getting to work on time.

A few weeks later, she also reported that she was growing hair in the bald spots on her scalp and that her fingernails were no longer splitting as they had been. "These are the strongest nails I've ever had," she reported proudly. After another couple of months, there were no longer any patchy bald spots.

Part Three

Women's Bodies Speak Their Minds

INTRODUCTION

It is paradoxical that a book devoted to encouraging people to look at their feelings should have a special section directed to a group of readers who generally are much more aware of their emotions.

For a hundred centuries of recorded history, women have been relegated to a second-class place in human society. It is only in the current century that they have attained a more equal status in society. Previously, women were a part of the fixtures in the home, expected to function in the home and to maintain their primary interests in the areas of the home and family. They were encouraged to stay in their place and "keep the house." So perhaps it is not so strange that this part should be such an important section of this book, because along with that conditioning, many women also learned to repress the expression of their true feelings about things.

The fact that the problems of women's sexual organs merit a separate section of this book will, I hope, highlight the need for women to be more aware of those internal emotional transactions indicated by their reproductive organs. They must learn to recognize unhappy feelings related to their sexual organs and learn to verbalize them. They must also learn to speak up to the men in their lives and voice their discontent so that their organs do not have to express it for them by becoming ill.

Men need women, and women need men, and both of them need to verbalize their wishes of what they want from each other to maximize both their satisfaction and facilitate their most complete integration into the master plan of which we are all a part. Further, women can lead the way for men to become more conscious of emotions, because men are generally less introspective and less aware of their feelings.

Women's normal awareness of emotions is enhanced by the upsurges of hormones that accompany the rhythmic cycle of menstruation. Women seem to be more intimately linked to the larger rhythms of nature. Their subtle awareness and appreciation of the small changes in the environment in which they live can make the difference between contentment and discontent, between harmony and uproar. Unconsciously, men seem to need women to help them more accurately answer the question How do I feel? and hope that the women in their lives are willing to help them answer this question.

Of course, the mere fact of women knowing how they feel is not always enough to keep their organs working well. If a woman feels unhappiness in the sexual department and does not acknowledge it to herself and/or to her partner, illness and malfunctioning of these organs seem to develop.

Generally, it appears that women have unhappy sexual organs because they have unhappy sexual relationships. Because they cannot recognize or express the dissatisfactions they feel, their generative apparatuses malfunction and manifest their feelings in various ailments of which only a few are examined here.

Often, these poor sexual relationships occur because their partners are unaware of their dissatisfaction. They can also occur out of insensitivity and carelessness, but most often the problem seems to be due to the male's unawareness of the woman's needs and desires. Nature furnishes the motive power by providing the sexual drive but frequently does not send along a book of instructions. The untutored male simply follows his instinct, which may satisfy him but leaves his partner wanting.

Too many women are reluctant to complain for any number of reasons. There may be a need for the woman to present herself as the completely liberated woman who, free of inhibition, can enjoy sex as easily and fully as her male partner. If she does not enjoy it, she is likely to take the blame herself, hide her dissatisfaction, and pretend that all is well. Or she may not complain as a part of a larger, personal pattern of repressing feelings of unhappiness. Then, there are a few women who still feel that pleasure for themselves is not to be expected and thus do not complain about lack of sexual satisfaction. Hopefully, this is a diminishing group. Other women hide their sexual dissatisfaction because they shrink from causing their male partners to feel inadequate.

Finally, sex is an uncomfortable subject for a great many people and the very relief that is needed, namely, open discussion of one's needs, is choked off by a widespread inability to talk about one's sex life. Most people seem to feel that they will be seen as inadequate or inept if they complain about sex or a particular sexual relationship.

But dissatisfactions between men and women are not limited to the sex act itself, which might be satisfying enough, but may be found in other larger aspects of their relationship. The man may be cold, distant, or nonrelating except in the sexual exchange. He may be adequate in intercourse but shares his attention with other women in such a fashion that his regular partner grieves at this affront to her bonding with him. Some men are simply more comfortable with other men and find themselves restless and at a loss for words with women, whom they regard as necessary for the sexual relationship but awkward for the comfortable exchange of ideas and general concerns.

The careless or thoughtless male partner oftentimes may simply be unaware. Frequently he is delighted to learn how he can enhance the pleasure of the exchange for his sexual partner. Even when he is unable to change his pattern, he can be complimented for "trying harder," and this can be balm to soothe his hurt feelings and raise the level of mutual comfort in the relationship.

Nevertheless, it is important to attempt to improve

unhappy relationships, particularly in the sexual area, because ailments resulting from the repression of sexual needs and feelings can be devastating to a woman's health, self-image, and feelings of worth. The emphasis here, as throughout the book, is, first, to pay attention to your emotions and try to recognize them early. Second, no matter how reluctant you are to admit how you really feel, try to be honest with yourself. Finally, share the feeling with other people, including your partner. The more you let out, the less your body has to express for you.

Should you, the reader, experience trouble with your reproductive organs, see your physician promptly. Many of these conditions can be serious and life-threatening. But if you can recognize the conflict that is making a particular organ behave as it does, you can often speed up the healing process by talking about it and perhaps avoiding a more serious illness.

LUMPY BREASTS

The breast is an integral part of a woman's sexual self-image. Her breasts are, in effect, advertising for her sexuality. The American brassiere industry is reported to take in 2.6 billion dollars annually, striking evidence of the widespread concern for this function. As evidenced in the animal kingdom, the essential dynamic of sex is simple: The female presents and the male aggresses. In human females, the breasts are part of that presentation. When the breasts are rejected as part of the sexual package, either by the woman herself or by her sexual partner, it is my own hypothesis that the breasts will eventually express that conflict or unhappiness by developing lumps, cysts, and even cancer.

Aside from my clinical experience, the hypothesis would seem to be in keeping with at least some of the demographics of breast cancer as defined by the National Cancer Institute. A higher incidence of breast cancer seems to be linked with higher-income groups, more education, age at first birth and/or childlessness, age, and overweightness. Traditionally, each of these areas could be seen to be linked to a reduction in sexual appeal and sexual activity.

Higher education and income in a woman, for example, could lead to more competitive sexual relationships, resulting in less attention to the breasts during foreplay or even a lessening of sexual activity in favor of work or other activities. Age and overweightness could be linked to a loss of sexual attractiveness, resulting again in less attention and caressing of the breasts during sex. Finally, late childbearing or childlessness could at its most basic result in loss of sexual attention for a woman on the basis of reproductive purposes.

These are all intriguing, though admittedly unproven, links between a most dreaded disease, some related disorders, and their possible connection to a woman's emotions and feelings about her own body and about sex.

Yet, in my practice, I have seen the link between sexually neglected breasts and the formation of lumps, cysts, and even cancer. If a partner was formerly quite attentive to the breasts and suddenly loses interest, yet the woman cannot bring herself to ask for those caresses, to determine the reason why, or to express her desire or feelings of rejection to her partner, the unhappy breasts may form lumps to express those dissatisfactions. Similarly, older women who have lost a sexual partner to illness, death, or disinterest may develop lumps or cancer as the body's expression of the breasts' dissatisfaction.

My personal correspondence with researchers about prospective and retrospective surveys on women's attitudes and experience and their possible relationship with breast cancer has not been particularly fruitful. Presumably, the idea is foreign to contemporary points of view. Also, most research on breast cancer is aimed toward treatment and cure, not cause. Perhaps, too, researchers are reluctant to embark on any survey that might lay a burden of guilt on women so afflicted as if to imply that the development of breast lumps or cancer was somehow their fault.

That is not the case at all, because our attitudes are usually not consciously chosen. It is not as though we decide to suppress our dissatisfactions or to be hesitant about asking for attention. These are part of an individual's learned patterns of behavior, not isolated decisions. My point is only that most of our attitude training does not reward assertiveness, and women's breasts seem to be suffering the consequences.

If nonproductive attitudes are a contributory factor in the formation of cancerous and noncancerous lumps in the breasts, it seems that counseling for marriage and sexual partners could perhaps save lives that are being needlessly lost. For those women without sexual partners or who have suffered the loss of a sexual partner, perhaps they will take the time not only to examine their feelings but perhaps to admire and indulge in the caressing of their breasts themselves in autoerotic activity.

Consider that it has been recently noted in the press that higher rates of breast cancer among young female inmates has been found to exist in a state reformatory for women. I wonder if similar statistics exist among other female prison inmates. If so, it seems like a harsh but made-to-order experimental setup for proving the link between sexual frustration or dissatisfaction and the development of breast lumps, cysts, and cancer.

CYSTITIS

Cystitis, or inflammation of the bladder, is most often seen in women. In the days when sex was deferred until marriage, physicians often encountered the condition in newly married women. At that time, it was sometimes called *honeymoon cystitis*.

In women, the urinary bladder lies above and in front of the vagina. The partition between the bladder and the vagina, including their respective walls, is about a quarter of an inch thick. It is therefore not surprising that many women have their first case of bladder inflammation after they have intercourse for the first time.

Cystitis can be the result of unfamiliar bacteria being introduced into the body or from the friction that results as the exploring penis stretches and rubs against the thin wall that separates the bladder and the vagina. The bladder becomes inflamed, and blood can leak from the wall, resulting in blood in the urine.

Further inflammation occurs when the bladder responds to the pain in the wall by going into spasm, so that the opening to the outside also goes into spasm. The urethra, or tube leading to the outside, becomes inflamed from the prolonged contraction, causing painful urination.

Once the bladder wall is inflamed, local resistance to infection is lowered. A stray germ can easily invade that tissue and multiply, and infection is established. Antibiotics are usually required to clear up the infection.

When the bladder is tensed up during intercourse, a woman is more likely to have her bladder traumatized by her exchange with the male organ. What is most likely to cause her bladder to be tense? Anger or aggression.

It is well established that the human, as well as dogs, foxes, and some other mammals, express aggressive urges with micturition, or urination. Traditionally, animals mark the boundaries of their territory with urination. Sometimes this almost ceremonial urination seems to be a way of saying "I can keep up with you," or "You can't get ahead of me."

In a therapy group, there are the talkers, and there are the quiet ones. If the talkers are allowed to monopolize the conversation for an unduly long period of time, the quiet members begin to squirm. If the exchanges are loud and prolonged, invariably one of the quiet members of the group will hop up in the middle of the discussion and hurry down the hall to the restroom. Upon her return, another member often will ask her, "What were you pissed off about?"

As the group builds up a history together, the quiet ones interrupt more often and run to the bathroom less. They say out loud that they are irritated, or "pissed off," and a suddenly contracting bladder does not have to say it for them.

Sally T., a thirty-three-year-old brokerage account executive, had been living with Ted for six years. She had come into therapy because of panic attacks. These had gradually diminished and were no longer a problem, but she had continued our sessions because she was not satisfied with her relationship with Ted.

"I have cystitis quite a bit, and I've noticed that it's most often when I'm pissed off at Ted. He's not a bad person, all in all, but sometimes he's selfish and won't admit it. Whenever I confront him about it, he counters by asking me if I would like him better if he were a wimp. I tell him he doesn't have to be wimpy just to have a little sensitivity.

"Last night when we got in from a party, I fell into bed—I was bushed. Not him. He got in beside me and started feeling me up. I knew he wanted sex, but I just wasn't in the mood. Ted always gets turned on after we've been to a party. He says it's because of being around all the women he can't have—and who can't have him. I guess I'm supposed to consider myself lucky to have him. Ha! Anyway, he was pushing, and I finally gave in just to quiet him down. This morning I had cystitis again. I called Dr. L., and he ordered some antibiotics without even seeing me because I've had it so often."

She continued, "I don't know whether I get it when I have sex and don't really want to or I get it because I have sex when I'm mad at Ted."

"Maybe both," I suggested.

"Well, according to you, I ought to tell Ted I'm mad at him and then I wouldn't get cystitis."

"Does that feel right?" I asked.

"Yeah, sort of. I don't know if I really feel some of this stuff or if you've got me brainwashed. I do hold back sometimes with Ted. I mean, if I lost him, I might not get another guy as good as him."

"Did you level with Ted last night about not wanting to have sex?" I asked.

"No, not really. I just grunted and tried to act sleepy, but he wouldn't quit. He can be pushy sometimes. I like that about him."

"So why were you mad at him?" I asked.

"Well, now that you ask about it, I just remembered why I was mad at him. I don't usually think of myself as being jealous, but when he was dancing with this woman, Mellie, she was all over him. I could tell he liked it. I didn't say anything to him about it, because I don't want to come off as jealous, but somehow it got to me. When he came onto me at home, I kept thinking he'd really like it to have been with Mellie. Pretty stupid, huh?"

"You can't help feeling what you feel," I said.

"Well, maybe I should have told him what I was thinking, so he could tell me it was dumb. Maybe I wouldn't be taking antibiotics if I had."

"Maybe," I agreed.

• • •

If you have cystitis fairly frequently, you may want to ask yourself if it is associated with unspoken anger or resentment, especially directed toward the man in your life. If you discover that you are angry or disappointed, you may want to try to let him know.

If you feel that confronting him is too formidable a task for you to handle at this time, try to share your feelings with a close female friend. If you don't have a confidante with whom you are comfortable, try a few sessions with a therapist. It may cost more than the antibiotics, but you and your bladder may both feel more comfortable in the long run.

DYSMENORRHEA

Menstruation is viewed by most women as an inconvenience at best and as a heavy burden to be borne with shame and indignation at worst.

As adolescents coming into puberty, young women often adjust with shock and disbelief to the reality of their part in the great reproductive cycle. Menstruation is handled with repressive customs in more primitive societies, where women are segregated as "unclean" during this time of the month, while some religions impose strict prohibitions about sexual activity during the menses and even the handling of foodstuffs.

Insecure males sometimes try to reinforce their sense of superiority with coarse jests and snide comments about this natural function. Many women attempt to compensate for their embarrassment on the subject as though menstruation really does mark them as inferior to males. By trying to cover this periodic indignity with "business as usual," they try to ignore their discomforts, worries, and emotions as well.

The harmful effect of any trauma of the spirit is exacerbated by feeling a need to keep silent about it. Many women feel they can't even complain to their sisters about their discomfort, and a vicious cycle can be established. It feels bad, they don't talk about it, and it gets worse. Because some women feel they have to hold in expressions of displeasure and discomfort, their emotions go underground and are expressed through their bodies with increased pain at the time of menstruation. Medically, this is called dysmenorrhea, or painful menstruation.

Kelly P., a twenty-eight-year-old cost accountant, had come into therapy for treatment of panic attacks. She had been able to reduce the attacks in number and severity after a relatively brief period of therapy, five or six months. One day she shared, somewhat shyly, that she dreaded monthly menstruation because of intense cramps that doubled her over but yet were not legitimate enough, in her eyes, to excuse her from work.

"I work with mostly guys, and they're not bad, compared with guys at a lot of places, but I can't very well tell them when I feel lousy, and I've got a big pile of work ahead of me. They just couldn't accept that. And even if they could, I don't want to be treated like a cripple just for being a woman.

"I was the only girl with four brothers, and they treated me okay. My father trained them pretty well about how men are supposed to treat women. They took up for me at school, and I always felt like I had 'protection'—more so than the girls who didn't have brothers.

"But the fact was, they were boys, and I was a girl. Do you have any idea what I mean? They had each other, and I was the odd one out. They could all go skinny-dipping out at the creek and I couldn't. It just never seemed fair. I guess I didn't think so much about it as I have since I've been in therapy.

"But it hasn't helped make my periods any easier. You said talking about things helped, but I still have a lot of trouble with my monthlies. Why haven't they improved?"

"Today is the first time you've ever mentioned it," I replied a little defensively.

"Well, it seemed sort of personal. I know you're supposed to be able to tell your psychiatrist everything that bothers you, but other than my family doctor, you're the first man I ever complained to about my painful periods. Do you think therapy can help me have less pain and trouble?"

"I don't know," I replied. "But it can't hurt."

Kelly's next period, she reported glumly, was as bad as ever. She kept talking about how being a girl in a family of boys made her feel like a minority member or a black sheep. She felt that being a woman automatically assigned her to an inferior group.

Even though logically she knew that her gender was "as good as" the other one, she still felt "outside." She joined one of our all-women groups and gradually got more comfortable about complaining in the presence of their acceptance. Much of the time, Kelly still felt she'd rather be a man, but as her intensity over the issue abated, she reported that her last period was "a piece of cake."

MENORRHAGIA

Sometimes, in the absence of any demonstrable pelvic pathology, a woman will experience excessive bleeding at the time of her monthly period. This is called menorrhagia.

Eileen V. was a thirty-seven-year-old delicatessen manager who had come into therapy because of recurring bouts of depression.

The oldest daughter in a family of four children, she was very close to her mother. During ten years of marriage, she had always phoned her mother daily. Her parents lived in the same town, and she and her husband, Don, were usually included in family gatherings. Her mother liked to say that when Eileen got married, they had not lost a daughter, they'd gained a son. Don seemed to feel comfortable with this relationship, because his parents lived in a distant state, and he saw them only once or twice a year.

As Eileen's therapy progressed, she became more comfortable with looking honestly at her feelings. She began to understand that her depression arose from a lifetime pattern of putting on a cheerful face and ignoring her discontent. Slowly, she improved her ability to notice small slights and unhappy events before they overcame her completely in the form of depression.

Her mother became ill with a particularly virulent form of bowel cancer. The prognosis was that she had only three to six months to live.

Eileen was devastated, but she tried to be brave "for Mom's sake." Despite my encouragement to weep if she felt like it, she showed minimal emotion. "The women in our family don't dissolve into tears," she said resolutely.

What happened instead was that Eileen began to develop gynecological problems, with profuse menstrual bleeding and severe lower abdominal cramping. "I haven't had anything like this since I was a young girl," she complained. "Every month I dreaded 'the curse.' I was knocked out for days before my period actually got started."

The symptoms progressed, and after trying various combinations of hormonal medications, her gynecologist recommended a D&C, or uterine curettage. When the bleeding continued, he told her they might have to do a hysterectomy.

"Don and I would like to have another child," she protested. "I'm too young to lose my uterus."

I agreed. I encouraged her to talk about her mother's illness and how she felt about the possibility that her mother, who had been so close to her all her life, might die.

"I hate it, and it terrifies me. It's so hard to act brave and cheerful around Mom when I know she isn't going to get well. I don't think I can go on without her. I love her so much." But she said she still couldn't weep.

I suggested gently that perhaps her uterus was weeping for her. "Maybe you're trying to bleed for your mother—if she dies, you'll die, too—or maybe that's what you're trying to say to her—or for her. Could that be?"

She dabbed at her eyes with a tissue and shook her head. The idea had been planted, and she looked thoughtful.

A week later, she came in looking tired and wan but with a new relief in her face. "My bleeding stopped," she reported. "I don't know if it had anything to do with it, but when I went home from here last time, the kids were in school, Don was at work, and I sat down and thought about how terrible it will be without Mom, and I began to weep. I sobbed and sobbed. I told myself it was all right, because we had talked about it. The next morning my bleeding stopped. I called my doctor, and he said maybe the medicine was finally working and that he probably won't have to do a hysterectomy. I feel awful but a heck of a lot better than I did."

Eileen's uterus was able to relinquish the job of weeping when she allowed her normal grieving apparatus to express her sadness.

The cyclic rhythm of the menses brings with it not only a periodic upswing of unfortunate comparisons with the other gender, but also upsurges of hormonal activity that increases a woman's keen awareness of her feelings. Usually viewed as an increased burden of anxiety and short tolerance, this time can also be seen as a period when Nature makes the woman hyperalert to her environment and more sensitive to her own emotions. In our ongoing quest for self-knowledge, any time of increased awareness can be considered an asset, not a liability.

ENDOMETRIOSIS

Endometriosis is the presence of little islands of uterine tissue distributed about a woman's intestinal cavity. These small foci of endometrium, the tissue lining the uterus, wax and wane with the menstrual cycle and can interfere with the movement of intestinal contents through the abdomen.

Anita F. was a thirty-nine-year-old sales manager of a jewelry store who had been referred to me by her family doctor. She had been diagnosed as having endometriosis, but in addition, she seemed to be depressed. Aside from her physical problems, she lacked energy and felt anxious. She suffered from interrupted sleep patterns and increased difficulty in concentrating on her job. During one of our initial sessions she said, "I just don't enjoy things the way I used to."

She attributed much of her anxiety and depression to the demands of her job. Her work experience was indeed stressful, but as she explored her feelings, it came out that she had experienced many previously unacknowledged pressures during her growing-up years that had ultimately conditioned her to be depressed.

Anita was the second child and oldest girl of a family of five children. The youngest child was the only other girl.

"My parents probably thought they were treating us all the same, but there was no doubt the boys had the best of the deal. My father and mother were second-generation Europeans, and they were sort of old-fashioned about a lot of things. The boys were not expected to do any work in the kitchen. They cut the grass in the summer and shoveled snow in the winter. My sister and I had to wash dishes, do the laundry, and clean house. It was generally understood that house-cleaning was women's work."

"How did it feel, being a girl, growing up in your house?" I asked.

"Well, sometimes it was neat. When Mom and Lucy and I would sort clothes together, it felt good sitting in a little circle in the basement. Then, at other times, when the boys were allowed to do things like drive the family car or stay out later than Lucy and I could, it didn't feel so good. We women were second-class citizens, and my mother encouraged Lucy and me to accept it, without ever saying it in so many words."

Psychiatrists have learned that people with depression frequently have unrecognized or unspoken conflictual feelings about their most significant other. Brooding dissatisfactions are transferred to the person from whom they traditionally would expect to receive support and encouragement—and frequently do not.

"How would you say you and your husband get along?" I asked.

"I guess you could say just that: We 'get along' and that's about it. We don't fight or argue about much of anything, but I don't get goose bumps when I hear the garage door opening either. He seems to get more excited about going on a fishing trip with his buddies than he does about going to Florida with me. We're glad we've got the kids, of course, but sometimes they're a drag, too, to be blunt about it."

Inquiries about the sex life of depressed patients frequently show a close correlation with their level of contentment. Sex acts like a barometer in the depressed patient. It could be said that a poor sex life causes depression, but it also seems true that depression contributes to a poor sex life.

"How would you describe your sex life?" I asked cautiously.

"It's just something we do, mostly," she replied without enthusiasm. "A lot of the time I can't do it with him because of my endometriosis. I get these god-awful cramps in my belly—and I mean all over my upper and lower abdomen—sometimes two and three days at a time. Willard is pretty good about leaving me alone when I'm having one of my spells. The doctor has tried me on several different kinds of hormones, and he says he may do one of these 'peekaboo' operations where they stick a light and a laser beam into a little hole in your stomach. But he says even that may not help; it would just make sure the endometriosis is what's causing all the pain I have. He told me it's as though my intestines are all stuck together with little bits of the lining of my uterus, or something like that. I guess I'm a mess."

I regarded Anita thoughtfully, thinking that this physical condition was one more reason to be dissatisfied with the role of woman, or was it the other way around? Did her unhappiness with her gender somehow cause the distribution of these aberrant tissue implants? "It sounds as though this is one more reason to think men have a better deal," I suggested.

"Well, it is harder to be a woman. When you're young, before marriage, you don't dare to have sex because you might get pregnant. Boys don't have to worry about that—it's always the girl's problem. Then, when you do get married, it's the same thing. The man doesn't have to worry about getting pregnant. I guess you could say I think men have the better part of the bargain, yes, definitely. Tell me, Doctor, now that I know this—and I've known it all my life—how is this going to help my endometriosis?"

"It isn't at first," I answered carefully, "but if you can keep talking about it and complaining about it enough, maybe your body won't have to complain about it so much."

"Well, I hope you know what you're talking about. I know my abdomen gives me fits, and if it doesn't get better soon, my doctor says I'll have so much scar tissue around my intestines that I'll get strangulated guts or something."

Anita did stay in therapy and joined one of our therapy groups, where she was able to vent some of her aggravations and dissatisfactions in the company of other women. She began to appreciate some of the uniquely feminine qualities that she shared with other women, such as their more accurate perception of emotions and their other awarenesses that the men could only wonder at but not comprehend.

Gradually her symptoms became less noticeable and less troublesome. She grudgingly acknowledged that some of the improvement was due to therapy, but she also thought the hormones helped. Probably so.

INFERTILITY

Mackey L. was a thirty-nine-year-old advertising executive who had come into therapy to deal with the panic attacks that terrified and even paralyzed her at times. She had discovered that the attacks were usually triggered by a new measure of her professional success and that she had much more trouble accepting the good things in life than she did adapting to the defeats and disappointments of her day-to-day experience.

In a therapy group, she had learned that such attacks were not at all unusual and that, in general, more people had trouble walking in happiness than slinking along in gloom. She learned that her panic had its origins in childhood where it seemed as though she'd be given a real comeuppance if she looked too happy but would be swaddled in comfort and consolation when she was unhappy.

One day in session, she settled herself into the chair opposite me, took a deep breath, and, with the air of a person who is about to make a serious pronouncement, said, "Doctor, Dan and I want to have a baby. We've been married twelve years now, and for the first eight years I was on the Pill, but I've been off it for four years, and I still haven't gotten pregnant. I'm going to be forty in two months, and it's high time if I'm going to do it. What do you think?"

"What do I think about what?" I asked, hedging somewhat.

"Do you think I just think I want to have a baby, but I really down deep don't want to?" She leaned forward earnestly.

"What does your gynecologist say?" I asked.

"He says to give it time. He says my tubes are open, my eggs are okay, Dan's sperm count is adequate, and it's a matter of letting nature take its course. He sounds like you sometimes. He says maybe Dan and I are enjoying being two people so much that maybe we don't want to be three. On the contrary, I believe if I didn't want to be pregnant, we'd probably have four kids by now. He said I'd better talk to you. So, here I am. What do you think?"

"I think it's hard for you or anyone to know what you really feel about a wide variety of subjects," I said. "Maybe we have to go back over your early years and see what comes up."

Mackey was one of five children. She had told me that her parents were married for seven years before they had any children. She related that they had finally decided they weren't going to have any natural children, and in desperation, they had gone to visit an adoption agency, where they were screened for preliminary suitability as adoptive parents. They were approved and told to go home and wait until they were notified that it was time to have a home visit by the social worker for the final approval.

Meanwhile, her father had cleared out a guest room in the house and had done some carpentry work to make it into an appropriate nursery. They began to tell their friends that they were waiting for their baby.

With some relish, Mackey reported that by the time the social worker finally arrived to make an on-site inspection of their house, her parents were able to announce "Thank you very much for coming to see us, but we don't need to adopt a baby. We're going to have one."

Mackey was the first of five children, and this family anecdote planted firmly in her mind the possibility that the attitude of the prospective parents had much to do with their success in the fertility endeavor.

Over the next few weeks, after she announced her decision to try seriously to get pregnant, she reported several dreams. "In this one dream, I was in our library, reading, and this cute little baby, a little girl, came in looking for me, and called me Mama. I realized with a shock that the baby was wondering where I was, and at the same time, I wondered why I wasn't taking care of her. She didn't say anything but just stood there with her finger in her mouth and looked at me reproachfully."

"How did you feel?" I asked.

"Guilty, I guess. I felt like I should have been in her room, watching her sleep or doing something motherly. She looked a little like Dan, but she had curly brown hair like mine. I thought to myself, she might look like an ordinary little girl to other people, but to me, she was beautiful."

"Did it make you want to be a mother?" I asked.

"Sort of. I don't like to feel guilty, though, so it was kind of mixed."

"What else happened?" I asked.

"Nothing. I just remember her standing there looking at me with that kind of reproachful look."

Next week, Mackey reported, "I had another baby dream. At least, I guess it was a baby dream. I was in this dune buggy—a big one—one of those that holds about six or eight people. I was driving and going down the dunes real fast when suddenly I got worried that the passengers might fall out. I looked over my shoulder at the empty seats. All the seat belts were fastened neatly together even though there was nobody in the buggy but me. I didn't have any passengers, and it felt good to have the wind blow my hair." All at once, she paused. "I don't want any kids, do I, Doctor? I'm too selfish to share my life with kids, aren't I?" She was silent for a few moments and stared at the floor. When she looked at me, her eyes were moist.

"I loved my little sisters and my little brothers, and we all got along like puppies in a litter—we were all pretty close together. But as the oldest child, I had to take care of them—a lot. Mom didn't mean to load them onto me, but it just came so natural—she always said I made the perfect little mother—that I just naturally took over a lot of their care. Lately, I'm beginning to wonder if I was as crazy about taking care of them as I thought I was. I know I loved my brothers and sisters, but—" Her voice trailed away, and she stared out the window.

"Let's quit for today," I said.

Over the next few weeks, Mackey did some urgent soul-searching and finally arrived at a position of comfort about her infertility. "Doc, you always say, your body never lies. Dan and I have talked about this baby thing quite a bit, and he says he doesn't care very much either way. He's afraid we'll be selfish old people if we don't have kids, but he says it's really nice that we can pick up and go away for the weekend whenever our schedule is free.

"Dan says—now get this—he says, why don't we just let nature take its course and let our bodies make the decision. If I get pregnant, that means we want a kid. If I don't, our bodies are pretty happy doing what we do without children."

I agreed that this seemed like a sensible decision. Mackey continued with her therapy for a few more weeks and finally left therapy with the parenting decision unsettled. Her other major objectives were well in hand, and by mutual agreement, it was time to terminate.

About a year later, I received a small pink envelope announcing the birth of a baby girl.

VAGINITIS

The vagina is a voluble protester when a woman is unhappy about sex.

When a woman is in the mood and is appropriately approached, the vagina moistens, swells, and becomes very receptive to the male organ. If, on the other hand, she is angry or unhappy, particularly toward her partner, the vagina ceases to cooperate. But, because women are highly adaptable to their partner's moods and attitudes, she may block her unhappiness with her partner from consciousness in the interest of a continued relationship.

Sometimes the first hint that a woman is unhappy with a male companion is that they are not able to enjoy what was formerly a good sexual relationship. The vagina complains so loudly that they are compelled to pay attention.

A gynecologist can treat vaginitis, or inflammation of the vagina, or other vaginal symptoms, but if the problem is the woman's attitude and feelings, as is often the case, even the best medical treatment is to no avail.

Your vagina always tells the truth. It says, "I like it," or "I hate it." Argue with it if you wish, even with the help of your gynecological physician, but it will always have the last word.

Alyson F., a forty-three-year-old registered nurse who worked on the psychiatric ward of a nearby hospital, came into therapy because of insomnia, inability to concentrate on her job, and weight gain. She agreed that this added up to depression and was eager to "get to the bottom of it."

"Many of the women I see who are depressed are having trouble with the man they sleep with. How do you get along with Bob, your boyfriend?" I asked.

She was thoughtful for a few moments and said, "I hate to say it, but Bob is almost too good. Anything I want to do is all right with him. We hardly ever disagree about anything, and if I like it, he thinks it's fine. I like him a lot, and I have trouble even thinking that my problem is him."

"How long have you been having trouble sleeping?" I asked.

"Well, about a year now. I really hated to come see a psychiatrist. I work with them all day long, and they're all right, but I wouldn't want to go see one of them—and I wouldn't want them to know I'm seeing somebody. I knew I had to do something, though. I've sat in on too many case conferences not to realize something was wrong. Besides, I almost gave somebody the wrong medication the other day, and that brought me up short. That's when I called your office for an appointment. I hope you can help me."

I thanked her for her confidence in me and said we'd have to work on it.

"I guess I should tell you, I also have herpes. The doctor said I should stop having sex, but I didn't want to, and Bob said he wasn't worried about it, so we have sex regularly. It doesn't bother him, but sometimes it hurts and burns on the inside and around my opening, so that we have to lay off a few days. I guess it's something I have to learn to live with. Do you think it has anything to do with my state of mind these days, or should I bother to ask?" She smirked a little. "You have a real reputation for being big on the body–mind thing," she added.

"Well," I said cautiously, "you came here for depression. Let's concentrate on that and see what happens with the herpes."

As the therapy progressed, it developed that she was unconsciously angry at Bob because he was too passive. An active, high-energy person, she felt guilty for being angry at him when his major sin was being "too nice."

"How can you get mad at a guy who always agrees with everything you say? I know he loves me, probably more than anybody I've ever known. I feel like an idiot when I think this way, but sometimes I wish he'd just blow up and say, 'For God's sake, woman, you don't know what the hell you're talking about. Why don't you shut up?' "

"So you get mad at him, but you feel guilty because he's so good you can't get mad at him?"

"Yeah. I guess he reminds me of my father. Mom used to nag Dad about anything and everything, and he'd never talk back to her. I can remember so many times when I just wanted him to hit her in the mouth because she deserved it, but he never even raised his voice to her. He was such a sweet guy. She didn't deserve him."

As the therapy progressed, Alyson began to see that by refusing to make decisions, Bob put the full load of leadership on her. In an effort to please her, coupled with his innate passivity, he "rode" on her energy and initiative. He trusted and relied on her completely, so much that she was smothered by his dependency.

As the months went on, she was able to gently point out to Bob that she would like for him to make some of the decisions, for instance, where they would go out to dinner. He was gradually able to see that letting her have her own way about everything was a kind of neglect and perhaps communicated a lack of concern.

This type of second-hand therapy was tedious and drawn out, but there was a gradual swinging back of the emotional pendulum. Bob actually showed up for a few joint sessions and was surprisingly apt at grasping the essentials of their unbalanced relationship. Somewhat defensive at first, he became cautiously enthusiastic about the process. "You're saying maybe I'm kind of a wimp, hey, Doc?" he offered in one session. I congratulated him on his courage for voicing that but assured him that in my opinion, he was more of a man than many other men who would have denied that their desire to please had gone overboard.

Not surprisingly, their relationship, which Alyson had originally described as "too good," became more solid, and her depression lifted. She also reported that the herpes symptoms had abated. A few weeks later, she discontinued therapy.

Minerva P. was a thirty-two-year-old librarian who had come into therapy for depression following the breakup of a four-year relationship with her significant other.

"I didn't get along well with him, really, for most of the time we were together. He was one of these people who always has to have the last word, and he was always right, even when he was dead wrong and knew it. In some ways he was a lot of fun, always ready for a new adventure, but when he was bad, he was a royal pain—really tiresome.

"I'm ready to give up men forever, or at least, I'm ready to 'celibate' the next few New Year's Eves with my cat. Men are just too darn much trouble. You can't trust them. They're all alike. Selfish and running over with ego—that cursed male ego—nothing personal, Doc."

She was silent for a few minutes. Then she went on, "I'm going to my gynecologist for a trichomonas infection. I know it's psychosomatic, but I can't psych it out. I've had it off and on for years, but this is the worst it's ever been. I used to get it when I was with Arnie. We'd have to lay off sex for a few weeks, and he'd groan about taking the medicine and say it was my fault, and then I'd blame him, but I really think it was us, not either him or me. What do you think, Doctor? It drives me crazy, it itches so bad."

"Tell me a little more about how it was with Arnie," I asked.

"What else is there to tell? Some of the time I feel like he was a male chauvinist, and I don't like to admit this—mostly, I guess I miss the guy." She flushed faintly and went on. "He was a little overweight—I used to tease him about his belly—but, well, I miss that big body of his. He was not very nice to me a lot of the time, but I even miss his being smart-ass.

"I sound like one of those cheap little hookers talking about her pimp. I wouldn't say that to anybody else, but bad as he was, he made me feel good most of the time, and I hate myself for admitting it, but I don't like being alone.

"Maybe that's why I itch so much—I want him, and I don't want to admit it. Does that compute? I'd be embarrassed to admit that to anybody down at the library. They know I'm upset about the breakup, but I think I have them convinced that I'm glad to be rid of him."

She was silent again, and she blew her nose softly. "I guess that's what the infection is all about. If it is, why doesn't it go away? Am I going to crawl back to him?" She clenched her jaw in a sudden burst of anger. "I'd see him in hell first."

She blew her nose again, louder this time. "Like it says in the song, 'What's a girl to do?' "

"Talk about it maybe?" I suggested.

Minerva was a determined woman, and she did talk about it, and eventually she decided that she didn't need to be talked down to just to keep a relationship. She gradually talked her way out of the longing for the emotional abuse of Arnie and men like him. She recovered from the separation and from the trichomonas infection and was able to go on with her life. When she met Sam a few months later, she was cautious, but she did "make a pretty good connection with him," as she said, and after a short time, she dropped out of therapy.

The vagina is so sensitive a barometer of the happiness of its owner that you may trust it implicitly. If your vagina is contented and functions well without complaint, things are good in your emotional milieu. If it burns, itches, goes into spasm, or develops an infection, have it treated to relieve the discomfort, but run a candid inventory of how you really feel about your partner or your life. If your vagina is unhappy, chances are you are unhappy, too, but haven't noticed or admitted it before. If you can figure out what is making you dissatisfied, avoid it, alter it, or complain as much as you can to as many people as you can. When you are back in equilibrium, your vagina will settle down and be happy, too.

Part Four

Screams from the Body

INTRODUCTION

A concerned parent is attentive toward his or her child. When a child is very young and murmurs a complaint, the parent tries to satisfy the child before the murmur becomes a cry or to attend to the cry before it becomes a scream.

Your body deserves the same kind of attention, for it is the only one you will ever have. It comes with no warranty nor guarantee. If it malfunctions, you cannot take it back or exchange it. When your body ceases to function, so do you. The point of including this part is to highlight the seriousness of the effect the emotions can have upon the body and hopefully enable you to avoid these disorders forever.

The messages in this part are full-fledged illnesses, and all of them are serious. That illnesses make a statement about the mind and emotions is a concept that will perhaps not be accepted by all who read this. Yet, I try to keep an open mind, and if anyone else has a more reasonable or logical explanation for serious illness, I hope I am not so immured in these conjectures that I cannot walk away from these concepts and embrace a new idea.

Meanwhile, even as I write these words, I find myself frequently experiencing my own share of the whispers discussed in Part 1. I feel good about it, for it keeps me from showing up so much in Parts 2 and 4, so far. As long as I keep on noticing the whispers, I won't have to listen to any screams. At least, that's the way I see it.

Let's now take a look at some of the things we want very much to avoid. Heaven forbid if the feelings described here jibe with your personal experience, either as an observer or as a participant. Please read on.

APPENDICITIS

Appendicitis is perhaps one of the most dramatic of the sudden illnesses. It is marked by malaise, vague abdominal pain, a slight rise in temperature, escalating severity of pain, and, in most instances, a localizing of the pain in the right lower quadrant of the abdomen. Rebound tenderness is the rule: Push gently into the abdomen on the left, then suddenly lift the hand from the abdomen. Instead of hurting on the left, the patient complains of pain on the right. The blood count shows a high white blood cell count with a "shift to the left" (i.e., many young white cells pulled out into the circulation), and the diagnosis is made. Generally, the patient is rushed to the operating room without delay to avoid a rupture, a surgeon makes the incision and removes the offending inflamed appendix, and after a short convalescent period, the patient is cured.

No one ever seems to ask, "What caused it?" It is generally assumed that it was something the patient ate, that the patient was too constipated, or that some infection or other settled into the appendix.

Years ago, I was struck by the fact that if appendicitis was mentioned in the patient's history, it was always accompanied by an extremely stressful event. It became a small hobby of mine: Mention appendicitis, and I perked up to ask "What was going on?"

Initially, the answer was always "Why nothing that I can think of." But a little persistent questioning on my part would invariably elicit a story of personal stress. Some of my favorites include the following.

• The little girl who was the darling of the extended family but was ignored when the clan gathered to celebrate her older sister's wedding. She moped unnoticed in the corner—until she was rushed to the hospital to have her appendix removed.

• The young Appalachian woman who moved "up North" and remained in her new suburban neighborhood, never venturing out until, after two years, her first visit to the "big city" for dinner and a movie. The excitement led to appendicitis.

• The little boy whose father said good-bye to him and his older sister and left to go to a job in another state, leaving him with his mother. He knew that Mom and Dad were going to get a divorce and he wouldn't be seeing his father again. He developed appendicitis that night.

I've found over the years that several other observers have noticed this correlation and tried to make a connection with concomitant stress and the occurrence of appendicitis. Their approach has been to look for events on the standard Holmes-Rahe listing of usual stresses. They found a correlation of around 25–40 percent.

Nevertheless, many stresses are internal, personal, and not of sufficient gravity to make the standard list. An event does not have to be defined as cataclysmic to be stressful, especially to the person who perceives that event as an explosive disruption in his internal feelings. My own personal surveys indicate a correlation close to 100 percent.

At one point, I conceived a grandiose questionnaire to be sent to all the persons listed in our local hospital records as having had an infected appendix removed. What was going on in your life? A family reunion? Was anybody leaving you forever? Were you or any member of your family in jeopardy with the courts or the authorities? Did you have or were you about to have a new experience you had never had before?

A computer search of the hospital records provided a gratifyingly long list of patients who had their infected appendixes removed. I was fired with the researcher's zeal, ready to add documentation to the connection between stress and bodily illness.

Alas, I ran headlong into the statutes concerning right to privacy. The research committee quite properly informed me the following.

1. I could not contact the patient until his personal physician had obtained his permission to have his records examined.
2. I could not subject the patient to this kind of intrusive, personal questioning.
3. I must guarantee the patient that his confidentiality would be respected in any publication of the results of the survey.

It became evident to me that I did not have the proper temperament to be a researcher, and so I abandoned the project and continued to conduct my "research" in the same informal way, that is, by questioning people I encountered in my practice who had had appendicitis. It continues to be a source of interest for me. Perhaps other workers with a formal organization and red-tape know-how will pursue this further.

In a group therapy meeting some years ago one woman remarked that she had heard me say that everybody I had ever met who'd had appendicitis told a story of a stress that was going on at that time. Ronnie, a fellow group member, scoffed at the possibility. "Ha! I had appendicitis two times, and I didn't have any stresses going on."

Mae, another group member, said, "How could you have it two times? Did you have two appendixes?"

"No," said Ronnie. "They weren't sure the first time, and they just watched me, and I was lucky it didn't rupture, because they decided not to operate.

"It was almost a year later that the second attack came, and when the doctor operated on me and took it out, he said that first guy really screwed up and said it was so scarred up I was lucky I didn't die with the first attack."

"What was going on when you had the first attack?" I asked.

"Well, I'd been drafted, and it was the night before I was supposed to be picked up by the bus to take me to boot camp. I got sick in the middle of the night, and when the bus came by in the morning, my mom had to tell them I couldn't go, because I was in the hospital. I didn't leave for the service until two months later."

"When did you have the next attack?" I asked.

"It was almost a year later. I was in the army by that time, and I'd had my basic training and all of my specialty training by that time. We were packed up and ready to ship out for overseas duty that next morning, and I started getting this terrible stomachache, just like before. I knew right away what it was, and the doctor said I was right. In the army, they don't mess around. They took me right over to the infirmary, got some captain out of bed. He got his crew ready, they got me ready, and he took out my appendix. My outfit shipped out without me, and I didn't catch up with them until four months later." Ronnie paused and looked around at his rapt audience, a dawning awareness slowly spreading over his face. "I'll be doggone," he said.

If there is a connection, what good is it to know about it? How can we avoid appendicitis or help our relatives and friends to avoid it? Perhaps, as we improve our individual awareness of stressful events, we can talk it out instead of having our body act it out with painful and life-threatening illnesses like appendicitis. If a painful, threatening, or disappointing event occurs in your life, you can give voice to your inner responses to that event. "This makes me very nervous (or frightened or jealous or lonely or sad)."

If we lose a spouse, a child, or a job or experience any severe disruption to our peace of mind or happiness, we must learn to recognize the enormity of the trauma and express it. Further, we must develop the ability to make loud noises commensurate with the enormity of the catastrophic feeling. Scream, tear out our hair, weep, and moan. Learn to recognize emergency emotions, and learn to make appropriate noises or fuss to share your unhappiness with others. Vent out, not in. That way, medical emergencies, like appendicitis, can be avoided.

ASTHMA

I can remember the feeling of awe I experienced as a medical student when I laid the head of my stethoscope for the first time on the chest of a patient having an asthma attack. I heard a sound I knew I would never forget. I knew that my patient, who was allowing me to listen to the low-pitched, violent screams in her lungs, must be undergoing torture.

During an asthmatic attack, each little pocket of air in the lungs suddenly becomes the bag of a tiny bagpipe. The entrance to the tiny bag constricts and lets the air out slowly, under pressure, and the tiny constricted opening makes a squeal like a bagpipe. Suddenly you are listening to ten thousand tiny bagpipes playing at once, like the famous Edinburgh Tattoo.

The myriad tiny cries coming from the little saccules, echoing along the converging airways in the lungs, are like a stadium full of little children who are faintly but urgently whining in chorus. Once heard, the sound is never forgotten and never confused with any other sound coming from the chest. Asthma attacks—and *attack* is the only word that seems appropriate to these episodes of sudden shortness of breath—often appear as though something triggered the spell of breathlessness, something that brought with it a feeling of terror, of abandonment, or screaming for rescue.

But this scream is not usually audible to the unaided ear. When air is sucked into the lungs desperately to scream for help, it runs into a conflict—a scream or cry is not permitted, because the air is trapped in each tiny sac at the end of each branchlet of airpipe within the lungs. Each saccule suddenly seems to seep (or weep) with increased mucus and fluid, and the constricted neck of the air sac becomes a microscopic vocal cord. The single, loud, urgent cry for help is shattered, or atomized, into thousands of tiny cries and held in the lung, audible only with a stethescope.

As with most symptom events of the body, the asthmatic attack seems to proceed like this:

1. Circumstance.
2. Emotion.
3. Physical response.

Symptom relief is effected by interruption of the chain of events between items 2 and 3. That is, medication that counteracts the chemical response of the body to choke off the air is injected into the bloodstream. The small saccules open back up, the cry dies down, and normal respiration is resumed. Currently, medication is available in small nebulizers carried by the patient for self-medication.

In the course of my psychiatric training, like all my fellow students, I was initiated into the mysteries of hypnotism. At first, to make true believers of us, we were hypnotized en masse. Later, we practiced on each other, and I, for one, was astounded at this newly acquired mystical power. I began to exercise this newfound skill on every patient who presented the remotest possibility that hypnosis would speed up or enhance their therapy.

As a resident on the psychosomatic ward, one of my patients was a man of forty-five who had periodic spells of asthma. When he would have an attack, I would hurry him into the pneumograph laboratory in a wheelchair. There, he would have a rubber-padded nosepincher gently placed on his nose to close off his nose breathing. Then he would pop the mouthpiece of the spirometer into his mouth, so that all his breaths, in and out, registered on a spiral cylinder.

With normal breathing, each breath registered as an even-sided little hill, like this:

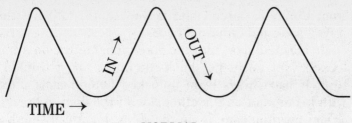

NORMAL

However, during an asthmatic attack, the front part of the hillock, instead of going up at the same rate it went down, rose up sharply as the breath was sucked in quickly, almost desperately. The second half of the hillock, in contrast, was long and gradual as the air fought its way out to the accompaniment of the wailing sounds of the ten thousand bagpipes, like this:

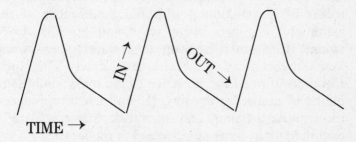

ASTHMATIC

I felt like a real scientist to have documentation of a medical condition. The patient would then be given an intravenous or intramuscular injection of medicine that would cause his breathing to revert to normal and end his asthmatic attack.

As he and I became comfortable with each other, it was possible to reexperience his prototypical asthmatic experience under hypnosis. When he was in a trance, I asked him to remember and describe what he remembered from childhood about his first attack. The patient slipped back to age five. The school bus let him off in front of his house, and when he ran up the walk to his front door, he turned and waved to the driver, who waved back and drove on.

He reached up to turn the doorknob, but the door was locked. Nervously, he shook the knob, but it wouldn't turn. It had always been unlocked before, most often with his mother on the other side of the door to open it as she saw him coming up the steps. Frantically, he began to beat on the door with his small fists, calling for his mother. No answer. He redoubled his pounding and his cries, which soon became hysterical screams. He pounded and screamed until he was exhausted. His mother was gone. Sobbing, the little boy slumped to his knees inside the screen door, his body engulfed in racking, muffled screams for the mother who had deserted him.

At this point, my patient, who was following all this replay of his childhood with the mouthpiece of the spirometer clamped in his teeth and his lips closed around it, began to register the typical quick-in and long-out breathing of the asthmatic attack. The stethescope confirmed the presence of the melancholy symphony of miniature screams. He and I had reproduced the emotional trauma and the attack that went with it, complete with spirographic record of the attack.

At this point, as the director of the little hypnotic drama, I continued: "Wait, there's a car driving up in front of the house. It has stopped. Your mother is running up the walk. Here she comes. She got held up and was so afraid this would happen. She's coming, here she is, she picks her little boy up and smothers him with kisses and tells him how much she loves him. She's so very sorry. How can she ever make it up to him? She loves him very much and will never let this happen again. Can you ever forgive her?"

The spirogram breathing reverts to normal. The attack is over. The patient gently sobs a little and awakens. He blinks his eyes and smiles.

I would like to report that when the patient left the

hospital, he no longer had asthmatic episodes. Such was not the case. My rotation of training moved me into the next subspecialty, and he was lost to my care. At that stage, I had not the training nor the experience to deal with a deep-seated characterological problem like this. Indeed, even after years of experience, I question whether I could treat it successfully.

The primary gain of the asthma attack seems to be the need to have the body express a sudden fear that the sufferer is unloved, abandoned, without emotional support. The stifled quality of the cry seems to betoken a fear that one is not supposed to cry for such things or that to do so is fruitless. The patient holds the fear inside the body, inside the breathe-and-cry machine, the lungs.

The secondary gain of the attack is, of course, the attention adults give to the child with the attack or to the adult whose child inside is expressing these terrible, unloved feelings.

The fear that one will not be rescued and will not be able to breathe is probably one of the worst sources of terror a human can experience. The victim is literally strangled, near to death, when all about her are able to breathe the air in which they both exist together.

Sometimes the victim dies in the midst of these states of so-called status asthmaticus, and so any asthma episode must not be neglected but treated vigorously, as is the case with any other life-threatening condition.

Still, the interaction between the primary gain, or expression of feeling, and the secondary gain, or cavalry-to-the-rescue, feed into each other. There is not a conscious awareness of this, but the pain-leads-to-pleasure (of the rescue) is a difficult cycle to break. I repeat, this is not a conscious transaction, and the possibility that it exists in every asthma patient does not mean that they should be made to feel in any way that they are causing this themselves. They are not.

How can the asthma patient be helped? If the aforementioned formulations are correct (and do keep in mind that the above is only one more of my own personal hypotheses), the patient may be improved by insight psychotherapy if she is an adult or family therapy in the case of a child.

Because patients do not usually come to me for treatment of physical ills, and I have never encountered a patient in psychotherapy who happened to be subject to asthmatic attacks, I cannot speak from experience of success. But it is a fascinating area and seems quite clearly to me to be yet more evidence for the connection between the emotions and the body.

ARTHRITIS

Movement in the human body is achieved through a series of hinges, or joints, that join the bones together. These joints are sealed and self-lubricated and are designed to last a lifetime. Under certain conditions, however, the joints become inflamed and painful, resist motion, and can even freeze or lock in one position. This is called *arthritis* (*arthro* = joint, *itis* = inflammation).

Most often the victim is unaware of any emotional conditions leading up to arthritis. His first inkling is the pain, then the swelling, the appearance of redness in the affected area, and, finally, the immobility.

Any motion or thought of motion involves the joints. You have only to think of squeezing a lemon, and you can feel the muscles of your forearm tensing, putting pressure on the joints in your hand.

If you have mixed feelings about the action of a particular joint, for example, the elbow, part of your wish is to move it in one direction, but part of your wish is to move it in the opposite direction. If both sets of muscles are pulling at the same time around the joint, it sets up tension in the joint, which tends to impede the circulation. After a time, it hurts, swells, and finally deteriorates, becoming fixed and locked.

Let's translate the above paragraph into feelings. Suppose you wish to punch a troublesome person in the nose (you want to extend the elbow). Suppose that person is your dear old father and you don't want to hurt him (you want to contract the elbow). Suppose further that these feelings are unconscious and unnoticed. If your father is very often in your feelings or you live in the same house with him, your elbow is tense most of the time. Yet, you aren't even aware of it until you notice pain, swelling, and redness.

As a medical student, I was led in with a group of other students to see a young woman who had arthritis in most of the major joints of her body. She lay motionless on her hospital bed, completely helpless, and permanently immobilized. One leg was partially extended, and the other was thrown forward as though to leap. Her hands were clawlike. She was covered only by a sheet.

The sheet was removed to expose her to our scrutiny, and far from being uncomfortable with our gaze, she seemed to enjoy the attention. After all these years, the clearest and most remarkable part of the spectacle was her apparent complete contentment with her own condition.

She was asked if she was in pain, and without moving her head (she couldn't), she joked in a squeaky voice, "No, only when I move."

Because all her major joints were frozen, she required complete care, including feeding, continuous frequent repositioning to avoid pressure sores, and, of course, excretory cleansing. Despite her complete immobility, all her soft organs continued to function. She seemed quite pleased to be where she was and had no complaints about her condition.

Without any psychiatric training at the time, I can still remember asking myself, What is going on with this woman? How can she lie there and smile so peacefully even though she is in this horrible condition?

Yet, her smile seemed genuine, as though she were glad to be there. And I couldn't help but wonder what terrible place she had left to find this an improvement.

My fantasy is that the young woman grew up in an atmosphere that clearly stated that no matter what she might want to do, there was a cautionary prohibition against it. Everything she did had the possibility of going or being terribly wrong. She was constantly on the alert to the possibility that whatever she did might turn out to be a disaster.

Finally she found the solution. Lock every joint into immobility, then you can't do anything—or anything wrong. No wonder she smiled so peacefully.

• • •

Lisa T. was a thirty-seven-year-old mother of three who was also a professional potter. An ambitious, energetic woman, she ran a small hobby store for other ceramic enthusiasts like herself, selling her creations and pottery supplies. Her customers bought supplies and brought pottery back to her for firing. She was able to contribute substantially to the family income and to afford extras like music lessons for the children. She was energetic about everything she did.

One day, in one of our sessions, she held up her left hand to show me the swelling in the middle joints of the fingers. "The doctor says I may have rheumatoid arthritis. I'm left-handed, and this is the hand I use to throw pots. Maybe the wet and cold of the clay is making it worse. My mother and grandmother both had arthritis. I guess it's my turn. Unless you think it's psychosomatic."

"I don't know. What do you think?" I answered.

"Well, I wouldn't have thought it was before I came here, but now, I don't know. I do know that when my hands get wet and cold, they ache like a toothache."

As Lisa's therapy continued, she became aware that although she enjoyed her ceramics work and her shop, she resented the fact that she had to work to help support the family. She was fond of saying that Don was a good husband and a good employee at his work, but she resented the fact that he relied on her to be the strong one in the family.

"Sometimes when he's acting dumb, I want to strangle him. He's a darling, but he's a jerk a lot of the time. He's always looking to me and saying, 'What do you think we should do?' And I can't help but hate him when he's weak and inept."

One day in a therapy session, Lisa said, "Do you know how you work wet clay when it comes out of a pug mill? You squeeze it and ball it up and slam it onto the table over and over. Yesterday, as I was working some clay to get it ready to throw on the wheel, I found myself squeezing the clay and imagining it was Don's neck. It was scary. I mean, it's one thing to say I'd like to strangle him, but it's another thing to act it out with a piece of clay.

"But you know something? Ever since I figured out that's what I want to do, my finger joints have been hurting less. My fingers haven't hurt at all since yesterday when I found myself strangling Don—in clay, of course. In fact, I was able to get my rings on my fingers for the first time in weeks."

Lisa's aggressive competence was working at cross-purposes with her desire to be taken care of. The struggle showed in the muscles and tendons around her competent finger joints. Part of her muscles wanted to work for Don and the family, and part of her muscles wanted to strangle him. The tension locked her fingers in a half-flexed condition, impeding the circulation, causing the joints to swell, and stopping her hands from doing any tasks at all.

Her joints were saying "Why doesn't he care about me and take care of me? Why do I have to work to take care of this family? I'd like to wring his neck."

Initially, Lisa was terrified when she discovered how intense her rage at Don really was. Yet, as she talked about it in therapy, the towering inferno of anger shrank down to a more manageable level. As she expressed it in words, her body no longer had to express her conflict for her, in tense muscles and joints in her hands and fingers. She learned to recognize anger and acknowledge its intensity, and also she came to terms with her husband's assets and liabilities. After all, he was lovable if not perfect. When the conflicting feelings became available for discussion, Lisa's arthritis was no longer necessary, and it went away.

If you are bothered by arthritis, you are probably a high-energy person who tries to be pleasant all the time. You probably know what you want, and when you don't get it, you try to smile and be cheerful anyway. That seems to work pretty well, except that you have swollen, painful joints—in your hands, in your hips or knees, or elsewhere, depending on what your conflictual feelings are.

To avoid arthritis and its symptoms, try being more open about what you want and perhaps a bit less accommodating. Learn how to complain if you don't like what's going on. For example, if your normal mode is to say "Oh, either one will be fine with me," say instead "Thank you for asking my preference. Since you asked, I'd really like [your honest choice]." People will be surprised at first, but they'll get used to it, and so will you. You'll be satisfied more of the time, and your arthritic condition will benefit. You don't have to become a curmudgeon, but try being less forcedly cheerful if you don't have to—and you don't really have to much of the time. Maybe you won't win the next election, but what good is that if you have to endure the agonies of arthritis?

EMPHYSEMA

When a medical student is learning how to do physical examinations, her proctor always advises her to make an estimate of the ratio between the lateral diameter of the chest wall and the anterior–posterior (A–P) diameter.

The cross-sectional shape of the normal chest, or thorax, is not a circle. It is an oval, with the greater diameter being from side to side and somewhat flattened from front to back. The usual ratio is near 0.7(A–P/lateral). The closer it gets to 1.0, the more likely the person being examined will be subject to emphysema.

In the normal breathing cycle, the lungs are expanded and then allowed to partially collapse with every breath to suck in air, then to let it out. The rib cage lifts and expands with each breath as the diaphragm flattens, first to pull in air, then relaxes to let it out.

The patient with emphysema is "puffed up" with a chest that never completely relaxes, as occurs in normal breathing. It is as though he (six or eight males to one female suffers from emphysema) is afraid to let all the air out of his lungs lest someone see him in a deflated condition and decide he is vulnerable to attack.

Most people's lung tissue is stretched momentarily when they take in a breath of air, but as every breath leaves, the lung tissue resumes its normal unstretched configuration during the relaxed exhalation phase. This is apparently not so in the person with emphysema. They seem to always hold in a little extra air, remaining in the semiexpanded condition.

In my experience, there seems to be two emotional forces operating in the breathing pattern of the emphysema patient. First, there is an above average hunger for love, approval, and affection, as with the asthmatic. Second is fear—of attack, rejection, or ridicule. Psychologically, he operates on the premise that if he is puffed up like a frog, attackers will beware and give him a wide berth.

He is likely to be a smoker. With cigarettes, smoke is supplied in profusion and creates the feeling of satisfaction, that is, "I may not be getting love, but I'm getting a lot of something." The cigarette has another important purpose in addition to filling up the hollow, hungry body of the smoker. It presents a facade of devil-may-care self-sufficiency: "I have my cigarette, I don't need you or anybody" says the cigarette. Of course, as with most poses, the stronger the pose, the weaker the poseur.

The cigarette smoker, like the ulcer patient and the gastritis victim, envisions himself as a hollow tube that wants to be filled up with love and mother's milk. When he inhales a lungful of cigarette smoke, he feels fulfilled, if not by love, then at least by a substitute. It doesn't make him fat the way those other big love substitutes, food or alcohol, can, and the nicotine stimulates and calms him at the same time. So he really feels he has taken in something tangible and comforting.

Does this mean that people get emphysema because they are hungry for love and affection? It does seem probable. The emphysema victim, most often a male, usually has a macho compulsion to deny his own needs. The emphysematous patient takes in great lungfuls of air and holds it in, trying to milk some satisfaction from this thin substitute for love. He can look full-bodied and extrahealthy or very self-reliant. But alas, this posturing is to no avail.

In emphysema, the air saccules in the lungs become distended, and the capillaries in the walls of the tiny sacks are stretched so that the lung tissue gradually becomes thinned and useless. The victim has to pull in more and more air with less and less oxygen exchange capacity. Finally, he has to breathe in pure oxygen in order to get enough of it into his bloodstream to maintain the body's needs.

What if your physician notices you have an increased

A–P diameter? Before your chest X rays begin to show the patchy areas of radiolucency that denote destruction of lung tissue, is there anything you can do to stop the onset of a disease like emphysema?

Traditionally, you're told to give up cigarettes if you are a smoker. Good idea, but psychologically and emotionally you're going to be hungrier than ever. What to do?

Psychotherapy may be an avenue that can help you become aware of your excessive craving for parental love and approval. If this idea seems totally unpalatable, then you may wish to run an inventory of your current relationships and think about how you felt when you were growing up. Were you coddled and cozened? Or were you always on the edge of the family circle, wondering what you had to do to be loved by your mother or father? Too much or too little early family affection seems to be a predisposing factor in the development of the kind of personality that may subsequently develop emphysema.

In any case, you are hungry for love and approval now, which is why you will want to reappraise your current significant relationships. Are you getting satisfying evidence of caring and concern? Do you receive many— or any—small spontaneous gifts of love and concern from your spouse or other?

Don't expect your demands to be reasonable. You want a lot—much more than you are getting and probably much more than you have any right to receive. Because you are so hungry—and perhaps a little petulant about it—you probably don't give as much as you hope to receive.

Suppose that you decide after considerable soul-searching that you do have a bit more than the average, unresolved childlike hunger for mothering. What then?

Simply put, admit it. But understand that on the page, it is not only simply put, it is downright simplistic. Most will have trouble recognizing the need in themselves for love and still more trouble admitting it. You may need some kind of psychotherapy to become attuned to your abnormal, raging hunger for love.

Does it help to be more self-indulgent? Well, a little self-indulgence won't hurt, providing you don't hurt others in the process. More importantly, if it is going to help your emphysema before it gets really troublesome, say to yourself "I'm hungry for love and affection. I want to be babied. I want to be coddled and spoiled. I never did get my fair share."

Even if you never get any extra mother love, saying out loud that you'd like to have it, writing it in your diary, or sharing it discreetly with certain friends gets it out of your lungs and into the air. Your body will love you for taking part of the load off your lungs by releasing it from your body. That can't hurt anything, can it?

HYPERTENSION

A rise in blood pressure is a normal, temporary response to stress. Physiologically, higher blood pressure seems to serve the purpose of driving more blood to the large muscles and is a part of the larger body response to our old friend, the fight or flight response. Our emotional response to an emergency situation is either fear (so you can run away better) or anger (so you can fight better).

Thus, higher blood pressure is the usual body response to a state of emergency. Physiologists monitoring the blood pressure of astronauts during liftoff, through remote reading instruments, know that their blood pressures may rise to 180/100 or higher until they are safely in orbit. After that, the blood pressures of these healthy young humans quiet down to normal levels.

People who suffer from chronic hypertension have responded to stress, but instead of the blood pressure coming back down after the emergency is over, they continue to exist in a state of emergency. Those with high blood pressure, or hypertension, operate as though they were continuously in the middle of liftoff. They cannot allow the blood vessels and the heart to slacken off and relax into a more restful, normal mode after the perceived emergency is over.

Sooner rather than later the system fails, because it is simply not designed to exist in this state of perpetual emergency. Stroke, heart attack, and kidney failure are all often related to hypertension—weak links in the body's support system. They give out, and the patient is disabled or dies.

If you are one of those people with chronic hypertension, who record a blood pressure above 140/90 most of the time, it may have gotten started due to fear or anger. Other victims include the so-called type A personalities—always trying harder, striving more intensely, or being unable to operate in a relaxed, comfortable mode.

If an inventory of your internal pattern indicates that you are chronically afraid, then you must become aware of your fear, examine it, discuss it, and try to separate yourself from it. It may be that you grew up being afraid most of the time and were not really aware of it. Why would you be? That's the way life was, and you had no real standards of comparison. Was uproar on the daily menu? Were arguments and fights a daily routine? Was the threat of ejection from your home due to nonpayment of rent a frequent possibility? Did you tremble inside most of the time for fear of incurring the punishing displeasure of one of your parents? Terror may have been your constant companion.

On the other hand, you may be afraid because of some more contemporary factor in your life. Does your bullying boss intimidate you? Are you having such trouble making ends meet you can't even think about quitting? You may develop high blood pressure as a result. You can tell some good friend that you are afraid of your boss, or tell two or three friends, which is even better. That will take some of the pressure down. The rule is, give voice to your feelings so your body doesn't have to do it for you.

On the other hand, your problem may not be fear; it may be anger. Stress and the effect on your blood pressure is multiplied many times if the anger is unconscious. And most chronically angry people who do have hypertension do not even know they are angry. If you find yourself angry, seemingly at random, and suffer from hypertension, there may indeed be a connection.

To let your tensions out and get them out of your body, blow your stack to a friend. To express your rage to several people is even better. The more you let it out, the less is held in. To explore in therapy the origins of your chronic anger is very important and perhaps essential to your long-term physical and emotional health.

In addition to chronic fear or anger, there is the type

A personality that is prone to hypertension. If you are somebody who has to go at a dead run while everybody else is strolling, you are likely to suffer from hypertension. Getting it out by talking about it won't be of much help here. "I'm a type A personality, darn it!" probably won't do a thing to lower your blood pressure.

There is help available, of course, both in addition to and instead of antihypertension medication. Yoga and/or meditation can help some people. More complex but even more effective is a combination of biofeedback, relaxation training, and group therapy as provided by the Meninger Clinic in Topeka, Kansas. Workers there have developed a regime of counseling, biofeedback training, and group therapy that allows individuals with hypertension to normalize their blood pressure, sometimes in as short a period as six weeks. They can probably put you in touch with one of the many people who have been trained in the Meninger hypertension treatment plan in your area.

If you have high blood pressure most of the time, but it is not yet serious enough to require medication or a course in relaxation training, consider a do-it-yourself approach. This will consist of talking to yourself and/or to your friends and trying to decide Am I afraid most of the time? Think about it. Perhaps it's the neighborhood where you live or the one in which you work that makes you afraid. Perhaps it's someone in your life who has you terrified. Try to figure out the why of your fear. Is your boyfriend a dope dealer? Are you afraid you'll both be caught? Are your children at risk? What about the IRS? There's a lot of these kinds of fears going around, and the effect can be devastating to your health. Maybe you need to cut off your association with a chronic fear-producing activity. Move to another town, find another boyfriend. Get your kids away from the neighborhood.

Anger is probably a more frequent cause of serious hypertension. Why are you angry? And who are you angry at? Your boss? Your spouse? The government? After identifying the source of your rage, try to get together with your friends, as in all of the examples above, and talk about it. Talk—you don't have to hurt anybody—just talk about it. It will help. Just don't allow yourself to stay in a state of rage. It will tear up your body if you do.

The personality is something that is not easily altered. Your chromosomal pattern is the start, and the "factory years" of zero to fifteen, when you were learning how to adjust to the world, leave a deep imprint on your attitudes. Can a personality be changed so much that your blood pressure settles down and relaxes into normal ranges? The answer is yes. But most people don't want to bother with retraining their habit patterns. It's easier to just take a pill twice a day and forget about it.

Whether or not you are aware of your feelings, do be aware that if you consistently show readings of more than 140/90, your high blood pressure could develop into a serious physical disability. Be concerned, and think about how those feelings you may not have noticed could be causing you a lot of trouble.

Follow some of these avenues to a healthier place, so you can let down, slow down, relax, and enjoy life more. That's really how your machine was designed to operate.

Try it. I think you'll like it better.

KIDNEY STONES

Urinary calculi (kidney, ureteral, and bladder stones) are caused when conditions increase the concentration and density of urine. These stones can occur when one is dehydrated or when there are increased amounts of the substances that form stones in the urine. Stones also occasionally form when the urine is not concentrated, but it has not yet been determined why this is so.

Generally speaking, small amounts of solids are always present in the urine, but they are usually carried out of the body in the liquid flow. When urine is retained, the solids are concentrated to the point of forming painful, health-threatening stones. Urinary calculi can be formed in the ureters, which are shaped like tubes, and the stones themselves have a tubular form. When there is severe chronic urinary retention, the stone can fill the whole cavity, or pelvis of the kidney, forming a stone called a staghorn calculus, an exact copy of the cavity. Usually though, stones are much smaller.

In terms of the body–mind connection, the formation of urinary calculi is a condition that seems to show up in people who remain in states of high tension or stress. These days, many people are under so much stress that they do not really relax even during sleep.

When a person is tensed up for a period of time, different organs, depending on her emotional climate, heredity, and other factors, seem to go into spasm. The normal progression of fluids in the body's containers (gland, bladder, or duct) is impeded, and a stagnation or holding in of the fluids occurs for varying lengths of time. As long as liquid moves in and moves out, there are usually no stones, because the small amount of solids are carried out as waste. However, it seems possible that it is during stagnation that these hollow casts form. When the stagnation is relieved, urine flows through the new cast, leaving the stone to harden in place, formed much like a pipe. Later, muscular peristaltic movements of the ureteral tube push the casts forward, and they cut the lining of the tube, causing pain and bleeding.

It is probable that the same principle applies to stone formation in other hollow organs of the body where calculi can be found—the gallbladder, prostate, lachrymal (tear) glands, and salivary glands.

That stagnation of fluids is the primary cause in the formation of stones does not appear to be in question by the medical community. Whether or not chronic tension is the root cause of stagnation is still, like many other ideas you will find here, a matter of speculation. For myself, I have little doubt that tension is the culprit, since my patients suffering calculi formation have uniformly been quiet, tense people.

Lois N., a forty-six-year-old advertising account executive, told me of the following exchange with a real estate saleswoman. "I had had her show me a few places, and when she showed me this old brick Colonial two-story, I really liked it. She knew I did, and I knew she wanted to make the sale. She was so anxious that I felt sorry for her. But I wasn't sure I could afford the place. I was trying to get her to go back and ask them if they would accept a lower price. You could see she wanted to but was afraid they wouldn't, and she'd lose the sale.

"We stopped to have a cup of coffee and to lessen the tension, we began to make small talk. I've know Marian for years and even bought another place through her. I asked how her kidney stones were, and she made a little face and said they bothered her from time to time. I knew she'd been operated on for them twice before.

"'The pain comes and goes,' she said. 'I'm having some pain right now, but nothing I can't stand. Yesterday morning I had a real bad spell. I could hardly walk, but I didn't give in to it, then it went away.'

"I primed her a little bit, and she went on. She began telling me about how she'd bought her daughter this wristwatch for her birthday. Marian told me her daughter took one look at it and told her she appreciated the thought, but she wouldn't be caught dead with it on. So Marian had to take it back. She'd really dreaded it—and then the kidney stone thing. Some coincidence, huh, Doctor?

"I didn't say anything, but I was thinking to myself, Maybe you don't know what brings it on, but I do. We talked about the brick house a little longer, and I called Bill about it, and he said go ahead and make the offer. So I did. Marian looked relieved, I signed the offer, and we said good-bye. Oh, yes, on the way out, I asked her how her kidneys were feeling, and she said, kind of surprised, they weren't hurting a bit."

If tension in the body leads to "puddling," or stagnation of body fluids, which in turn leads to stone formation, then how do we avoid the levels of tension that cause our involuntary muscles to clamp down and the fluid flow to stop?

It is not a simple task. It requires attention to our state of mind on a regular, ongoing basis until we feel comfortable and relaxed the majority of the time. Yoga, meditation, biofeedback, and most relaxation procedures of that type can help anyone to avoid the kind of accumulated tension that causes us to clamp down the valves of the body's fluid flow that leads to the formation of stones.

Psychotherapy, especially group therapy, can be very helpful in training you to release tensions. Any practice or therapy that increases your awareness of what makes you comfortable or uncomfortable will undoubtedly help you to be more relaxed. Increased relaxation will cause the muscles that open and close your body's disposal systems to open and close smoothly and regularly, avoiding the formation of stones.

Certainly reading books like this can help you to be more aware of what you like and move toward it. When you are in the pleasure zone, your body is comfortable, untensed, and probably in a non-stone-forming condition. On the other hand, if this book helps you pay more attention and be more aware of what you don't like, you can work to avoid those situations that make you tense. If that's impossible, then you can learn how to complain constructively so as to let out the tension from inside your body. As your sympathetic nervous system (it does sound as though it's on your side, doesn't it?) relaxes into a comfortable rhythm of gently opening and closing the smooth muscle valves, your fluids will flow where and how they should. Result: no stones.

In your search for serenity, leave no stone unturned, and hopefully you will also leave them unformed.

YOU ARE WHAT
YOU FEEL

After reading this book, we can undoubtedly see there is one more axis along which to divide people's attitudes. We have prolife versus prochoice, liberals versus conservatives, those who believe in UFOs and those who don't. We also have those readers who believe that emotions can and do affect the body's health and those who think body and mind are independent of each other.

Group A is the people who find it interesting that with every emotion, there are changes that occur in the body. It seems apparent to them that mind and body continuously interact.

Group B is the people who will have none of it and insist the mind is the mind, the body is the body, and never the twain shall meet. Group B people attribute illness and health to spontaneous chemical changes that begin inside the body and must be corrected by appropriate medicines to restore health. To this group, a sigh is just a sigh—it has nothing to do with getting sick.

Group B people prefer to take medication for their hypertension, their infections, or their colitis rather than to "get into all that psychological jazz. You psychiatrists are all alike. Everything that happens to me is my own fault. If I would only think right, I would feel good. I'm not buying it. What is all this nonsense about getting in touch with your emotions so your body can be healthy? Disease is a happenstance or fate or bad luck. If you're gonna live, you're gonna live; if it's your time, you'll die."

Group A says "Maybe bad things do happen to you, including illness. But maybe you feel bad first, and your body reflects the bad feeling and allows your immune system to stop functioning, making you more susceptible to infection. Cancers happen, but maybe they are a powerful statement of the body's despair. Chronic anxiety leads to chronic tension of the voluntary muscles and causes aches, pains, and even arthritis. Tension can also cause spasms of the involuntary muscles in the walls of blood vessels, bladders, and secretory glands, so that thromboses [clots] and calculi [stones] are formed. And maybe tension is the real culprit in high blood pressure, strokes, and heart attacks."

Assuming that perhaps Group A is correct, how do we stay in the happy zone? What do we do about the inevitable disappointments, rejections, anxieties, and disparaging words, which are so much a part of life yet perhaps lead to the dis-ease of the body?

Does talking about it lessen our fears? Does it do any good to know that we are sad and disappointed? If we share our burdens with a friend, do we feel better? Will it help lessen the pressures on our body systems so that we can become healthier and stay that way?

I think so.

In my first week of medical college, my fellow students and I were treated to a lecture by a visiting celebrity physician, the world-renowned diagnostician and gastroenterologist Dr. Walter Alvarez, who at that time was the editor of *The Journal of the American Medical Association*.

In a dramatic gesture, he picked up a three-inch-thick chart from among several lying on the table before him and waved it around for all of us to see. "My job is to make a diagnosis of patients with thick charts like this, the ones who have been seen by dozens of doctors. These patients have so many symptoms that nobody can decide what is wrong with them.

"I'll share a trade secret with you. I always read the whole chart, but I know the diagnosis as soon as I see a chart this size. It's always the same—nerves. Never forget that. Nerves."

I haven't.

Everything that has ever happened to you is recorded in your body, in that computer that never forgets. Every event that you experience impacts upon you with good feelings or bad. If something gives you a good feeling, every cell in your body is favorably affected and benefits therefrom. If something happens that makes you feel bad, then your body feels bad, and once more, every cell in your body is influenced in a harmful or unhappy way.

Whether you experience one large bad feeling or an accumulation of small bad feelings and are unaware or unable to give expression to those feelings, your body will respond with pain, inflammation, cramping, or other symptoms of illness. If you have more unhappiness than you can handle, your body will give up the struggle, and you can die. The unfortunate fact is, when you become ill, most of the time you didn't even notice the original bad emotion that led to your physical illness.

Still, in the course of your life, you will most likely experience a series of bad feelings interspersed with a series of good feelings. Good health on the whole seems to depend on the relative intensity of those feelings—how good the good and how bad the bad. Stronger feelings cancel out less intense ones. Norman Cousins noted that when he was ill, he could expose himself to a series of good stimuli (funny movies that made him laugh) and was able to counteract his bad feelings and become well. Another factor in his recovery was the opportunity he took to take charge of his own treatment and work his way out of a feeling of powerlessness, which may have made him ill in the first place.

Although each one of us is a separate individual, in a sense, we are part of something larger—the community of people with whom we live and interact and who make up our world. In the nourishing atmosphere of that community, we talk, laugh, console, and share our feelings, so that we all partake of the happiness and unhappiness of our group members. If we are experiencing unhappy feelings as individuals, then the sooner we can share them with the rest of our fellow humans, the sooner the burden of our unhappiness dilutes, spreads around, and lessens.

If you would be happy, have happy experiences. Gravitate toward them, prolong them if you can. Remember, just as sharing your unhappiness dilutes unpleasant feelings, sharing your happiness with others increases it.

To avoid illness, then, be alert to how you feel all the time. The moment you experience a bad feeling, get it out of your body by acknowledging it and then by letting it out—in words, cries, tears, journal writings, and especially by telling your fellow human beings about the feeling. Never let the bad feelings accumulate inside yourself so that your body has to do your complaining for you.

If you have read some, most, or all of the foregoing, this is what I hope you have by now considered:

• Your emotions are constantly registering pleasant feelings, unpleasant feelings, or a mixture of the two. For every feeling, there is also a body response right along with the emotional response.

• Most of the time, we accept pleasant feelings without comment and, indeed, without particularly noticing. If we are in the good or pleasant mode, the body functions well, and the machinery runs smoothly.

• If we are in the unpleasant mode, we frequently don't notice that either. If we continue in the feel-bad mode for very long, even though we may not consciously notice it, the body does, and it begins to register unpleasant symptoms. We call this illness.

• It is possible to head the bad symptoms off at the pass, notice them at the first whisper of bodily discomfort, and perhaps figure out what unpleasant emotional experience we have just had, which is being communicated by a bodily symptom.

• If we notice an emotion, we call it a feeling. If we can talk about the feeling, share it with the world and with others, most of the time, it will magically abate. As soon as we begin to talk about it, the organs that have been expressing an unhappy feeling for us can relax and resume their pleasant, normal functioning. We can then remain well and happy, which, it turns out, are probably one and the same.

• Any time your body has a sudden, unexplained new feeling, it is probably a response to an emotional perception. With continuing attention and practice, you can figure out what emotion your body is expressing and release it. Complain, whine, grouse, cry, accuse, growl, grumble, lament, moan, and grieve. Avoid suffering in silence at all costs.

The medical profession has made enormous strides in its understanding of the functioning of the human body in sickness and in health. Illnesses that were inevitably fatal a generation ago, are treated and cured routinely now. The next great frontier of medical research may be to clarify the hazy connection between our emotions and our bodily functioning. Perhaps researchers will pay increasing attention to the possibility that the body follows the emotions' lead.

Finally, to be healthy, be happy. Given the choice, move toward pleasure as often as you can. We all must accept responsibility and do our share of the world's work, but try to do it in a way that gives maximum production with minimum pain. Between your periods of work, sandwich some relaxation and pleasure. A minimum amount of happiness is not just a luxury, but a necessity.

Pain, sadness, and unhappiness will occur, of course. "Be happy" does not mean covering up your pain with a smiling face. It means let out the pain by talking about it. As unhappiness is released by sharing it with others, we feel better. And if we feel good enough, this is happiness. And happiness is what keeps us healthy in the end.

INDEX

breathing, 116, 117, 184
breathing problems:
   asthma, 173–78
   emphysema, 184–87
bursitis, 96

calculi, urinary, 19, 192–95, 197
cancer, 11, 14, 18–19, 28, 59, 196
   breast, 137–38, 139
Cannon, Walter, 34
capillaries, *see* blood vessels
carpal tunnel syndrome, 61
catecholamines, 33
cerebrum, 29, 33
choking and coughing, 48–50
cigarette smoking, 185, 186
clots, blood, 197
cold hands and feet, 20, 37, 60–62
colds, 11, 56, 70, 113–15
colitis, 73
constipation, 74–76, 78, 168
coughing, 48–50
Cousins, Norman, 198
crying, *see* tears
cystitis, 140–43

depression, 25, 147, 150, 158, 159, 161
   sexual relationships and, 151
   see also sadness and unhappiness
diarrhea, 73
digestion, 25, 26, 28
   see also bowels; stomach
dry mouth, 63–66
dysmenorrhea, 144–46

eczema, 123, 125
embarrassment, 44, 46, 47
emotions:
   awareness of, 11, 12, 13, 14, 19, 24–26, 28, 33, 36–37, 38, 43, 199, 133–34
   brain and, 29–32, 33
   chemical changes caused by, 33–34
   conflicting, 48, 49, 50, 182, 183
   coping strategies and, 25, 26–27

duality of, 33–39
   expression of, 24, 34–36, 37, 38, 85, 198, 199–200
   illness related to, 10–14, 18–21, 23–28, 38, 43, 85, 167, 196–200
   immune system and, 27–28, 59, 196
   importance of awareness of, 24–26
   irrationality of, 89
   neuroses and, 29–32, 35, 36, 38, 85
   physical manifestation of, 24, 25–26, 33–34, 37–39, 196
   social conditioning and, 24, 31–32, 34, 35
   unique physical expressions of, 19–20
   unnoticed and suppressed, 11–12, 13, 14, 19, 23, 24, 25, 31–32, 34–35, 36–37, 43, 74–76, 198, 199
   women's awareness of, 133–34
   see also specific emotions
emphysema, 184–87
encephalins, 59
endorphins, 59
eyes, 67–69
   itchy, 68–69
   twitches and, 23, 67–68
   see also tears

fear, 37, 197
   and cold hands and feet, 60–62
   colds and, 114, 115
   dry mouth and, 63–66
   emphysema and, 184
   eyes and, 67, 68
   hypertension and, 188, 189
   see also nervousness
feelings, *see* emotions
feet, cold, 20, 37, 60–62
fertility problems, 154–57
fight or flight response, 33–34, 63, 67
   blood pressure and, 188
   blushing and, 44, 45, 46

ABOUT THE AUTHOR

Dr. Rush lives and practices psychiatry in Middletown, Ohio. He interrupted his medical-school training to study for two years at Oxford University in England on a Rhodes scholarship. He obtained an M.A. in the Final Honour School of Animal Physiology.

After medical school, he practiced general family medicine for five years. He left his practice and returned to school to study psychiatry, so that he could better understand why his patients became ill when under stress. Since then, he has practiced only psychiatry.

Dr. Rush has a son and a daughter. He and his wife live on the edge of a golf course, even though neither he nor she plays golf. "It makes a fine big front yard, and I don't have to cut it," Dr. Rush explains. "Besides, looking out the window at so many people having fun makes me feel good. Happiness is a contagious condition."